NUTRITIONAL SUPPLEMENT USE
FOR AUTISTIC SPECTRUM DISORDER

By Jon B. Pangborn, Ph.D.
(With lots of help from Chris!)

Autism Research Institute
San Diego CA
2012

DISCLAIMER

The author, Jon Pangborn, Ph.D., F.A.I.C., is not a medical doctor or physician. He does not diagnose or treat disease. This book is only intended to share knowledge and information gained from experience and research. Dr. Pangborn has been affiliated with the Autism Research Institute for 30 years, and in the past, he practiced as a licensed and certified nutritionist (IL).He is a parent of an individual who was autistic as a child and who continues to have special needs. He is retired from all consulting and from all professional relationships with laboratories and supplement manufacturers.

Nothing within this book is intended to substitute for a direct relationship with a medical doctor or health professional qualified to give medical advice. The reader is encouraged to always seek such advice from a licensed health professional.

This book is dedicated to physicians and scientists who pioneered nutritional therapy for environmental illness and who opened my eyes to something that is going very wrong with our world:

William H. Philpott, MD
Thomas L. Stone, MD
Marshall Mandell, MD
William J. Rea, MD
Theron Randolph, MD
Abram Hoffer, MD
Carl C. Pfeiffer, MD
Herbert J. Rinkel, MD
Linus Pauling, Ph.D.
Roger Williams, Ph.D.
Dwight Kalita, Ph.D.
Bernard Rimland, Ph.D.

And many others who are not listed.

ACKNOWLEDGEMENTS

This book would not exist had it not been for the diligent efforts of my wife, Christine Pangborn (Chris), who shares with me the desire to help other families deal with the tragedy of autism. Chris keyed in the entire text and created the tables and diagrams.

Many thanks to Sidney MacDonald Baker, MD for reviewing the manuscript and for his three decades of friendship, support and guidance.

We are most grateful to Anne van Rensselaer for her splendid editing job, which she provided gratis. Anne is the mother of Jane Johnson, a member of the Board of Directors of the Autism Research Institute, San Diego.

Also, sincere thanks to Leah Cooper for a beautiful job of formatting and final editing.

Thanks to Steve Edelson, Ph.D., ARI Director, who waited patiently for me to write this so that he could get it published by the Institute.

TABLE OF CONTENTS

PREFACE

Chris and I became the proud parents of our first child, a son, in 1967. That same year, I received my Ph.D. in Chemical Engineering and I (we!) went on active duty with the US Air Force. Three years later, we had to face the realization that our son was autistic – a behavioral diagnosis made by psychologists at Sutter Memorial Hospital in Sacramento, California. We've been wondering, thinking, studying and researching autism since that time, over 40 years ago.

In 1967, Dr. Bernard Rimland was way ahead of conventional wisdom in his efforts to understand autism. He established the Institute for Child Behavior Research in San Diego and nurtured it as director until his passing in 2006. Bernie and I met in 1980 at a Clinical Ecology meeting. Clinical Ecology is the medical study of how environmental factors contribute to disease and of interventions that may alleviate such diseases. Bernie and I wound up at the same place for the same reasons – we suspected that our toxic environment is where many of the answers to autism will be found.

Bernie realized the connection between environment and autism very early on. The Autism Research Institute, which the ICBR eventually became, has a video production that commemorates his views, discoveries and accomplishments. That video (or DVD) contains a clip from an interview that Bernie gave in the 1970s in which he states his findings about the cause of autism. It is not due to cold, unloving or indifferent parents. It is due to environmental factors that work with genetic predispositions to cause a condition of deficient speech and lack of interaction with others and with the environment.

Many researchers in mainstream medicine have tried to establish autism as a primarily genetic fault. In fact, this is rarely the case. Even though many years and many millions of dollars have been spent to prove this hypothesis, the results have been meager and frequently inconsistent. Do you remember hearing about how, in times past, coal miners used to take a canary down into the mine with them? If toxic gases were present, the canary would die. When that happened, the miners would evacuate as quickly as they could, before they died, too. Canaries are genetically and biologically more susceptible to toxic gasses than humans. But, when they died in mines, it didn't mean that there was something wrong with the canaries – it meant that something was wrong with the mine environment.

ARI and the Defeat Autism Now effort (1995-2010) diligently pursued that concept - the vast majority of autism is the result of toxic or infectious stressors propelling otherwise subclinical imperfections in metabolism into a pathologic condition. Often insidious in onset, autistic traits do not become apparent until the child is at the stage of development where neuronal networks in the brain are learning to communicate with each other and with the outside world. Unfortunately, the toxic soup we live in is getting worse and worse, and so is the incidence of autism.

Genetic makeup is fixed. However, some of genetic expression is environmentally determined, and some of that is due to inflammation. If you can relieve inflammation, you may be able to improve the autistic condition. While that's often a difficult task, once done it facilitates improvements that may be gained through relational therapy, special education, persistence with patience, and lots of love. But if you don't relieve persistent stressor-caused problems, like inflammation, then your efforts are much less likely to be successful. This book is about how to relieve acquired stressors with nutritional strategies. It's also about why nutritional supplements alone won't get the job done.

HOW TO USE THIS BOOK

The INTRODUCTION and BACKGROUND sections serve to orient you to the complexity of the problem. Please do not expect one type of therapy to bring about remission or even notable improvement. Should that happen, you'd be unusually lucky. For almost all with autism or autistic spectrum disorder, significant improvement requires: purifying the habitat and environs, dietary intervention, use of nutritional supplements, medical interventions, relational therapy and special education. What's described in this book is one tool in the toolbox that you'll likely need to do the job. And, unfortunately, there are some who can't be significantly helped no matter how hard we try.

As you go through INTRODUCTION and BACKGROUND, you'll find that there are prerequisite problems to deal with before doing trials of nutritional supplements. Please do not ignore these tasks; they are essential to success. As with everything in this world, there are rules to follow if you want the best outcome. Nutritional supplement use is no exception. There are six rules to follow, and I've provided a dozen "don't-dos" which are common pitfalls to success.

Next comes what you're probably most interest in – the INTERVENTION SCHEDULE for nutritional supplement trials. It's in five successive parts that I've named "tiers". Yes, there are other orders for doing what I've outlined. If you have a very experienced coach, you may be able to change the order of what's done ahead of or after something else in this schedule. But I'm assuming you don't have such a coach. So, I've provided an order of intervention that is, in my experience, least likely to cause problems.

The INTERVENTION SCHEDULE does not include specific information about the listed nutrients. That information is contained in the following part – TECHNICAL INFORMATION ON SUPPLEMENTAL NUTRIENTS. That section tells you about indications for, how much to use, and what might be behind problems with use. When it comes time to do trial use of the next nutritional supplement, find the text on that nutrient in the TECHNICAL INFORMATION section and read it. There's more nutritional chemistry in this section than most of you will need to know, so concentrate on the "Indications of Need" and the "When and How Much" parts, and leave the rest to those who want the details. Nutrients in the section are ordered alphabetically, not in the order described in the schedule.

There's an APPENDIX section with several parts – environmental junk to avoid, nutrient cooking information and how the circadian rhythm influences supplement use.

Following this, there's a GLOSSARY which I hope will help with some of the nutritional biochemistry language that unavoidably slips into an effort like this.

A thought:

Life is what happens while you're making other plans.

– John Lennon

INTRODUCTION

Biologically, autism isn't one disease; it doesn't have just one underlying genetic predisposition; it doesn't have just one acquired stressor or instigating trigger; it doesn't have only one curative strategy; and it may not be curable or reversible. However, there are over 27,000 parents who have reported improved abilities and behaviors in their autistic children following use of nutritional supplements. Specific information on this is available from the Autism Research Institute (ARI), 4182 Adams Avenue, San Diego CA 92116, 1-619-281-7165, www.autism.com. Parent opinions on types (not brands) of nutritional supplements are compiled and updated every couple of years on one sheet of paper, ARI Publication 34. The latest edition of this piece of paper costs $1.00 to get by US mail, or you can download it (free) from the ARI website. The latest edition I have, as of this writing, is included here in the Appendix.

A Spectrum of Disorders with One Name

Because of the extreme variability in traits and severity, the name for the disorder, "autism", has in recent years been modified to autistic spectrum disorder, "ASD". That variability makes our job − nutritional intervention − more complicated. What worked for Johnny down the street may not work for your child. I don't have a recipe for nutritional success − and there's no guarantee that nutritional supplements will help. I make no promises. But, the odds are in favor of benefit. With melatonin use, for example, 66% show sleep and behavioral improvements. That's according to 1687 parent reports to ARI (as of March 2009). And while there's no set protocol for nutritional intervention, there is a schedule for trying various interventions − what could work initially and what is best put off until later. You will learn about that schedule by reading this book. But before we get into those details, let me tell you about my concept of ASD. This is important because the strategies described for nutritional intervention are based on this concept.

Causative Stressors for ASD

Relatively few ASD individuals are that way only because of an inborn error of metabolism, that is, relatively few are hard-wired for ASD by genetics. Excluding phenylketoniuia (PKU), there are at least two dozen rare but severe inborn metabolic diseases that may feature ASD or at least some autistic traits. Some of these diseases are due to metabolism

1

errors in energy delivery to brain cells, such as defective creatine formation or transport. Other genetic problems involve the base molecules of RNA and DNA which also have energy-transfer duties (adenosine, guanosine). Inborn errors to neuronal growth and structure and to neurotransmitter functions can be at fault as well. I believe these kinds of genetic defects have always been with us and that today, their contribution to the total incidence of autism is minor. When I refer back to the writings of early investigators (1950s, 1960s), the total incidence of autism was thought to be about 4 or 5 in 10,000 births. I credit the geneticists of those earlier times for recognizing that, back then, genetics played a relatively major causative role. And, back then, maybe they were missing half of autism due to incomplete reporting. So, let's double the historic incidence to 10 in 10,000 and then ask, what is causing all of the rest? What is causing the additional 90 more per 10,000 that we now have – for a total of roughly 100 in 10,000 births that become ASD kids?

As portrayed by Paul Shattock, Director of the Autism Research Unit in the United Kingdom, the ability of the human population to withstand toxic and infectious stressors follows a bell-shaped curve, most likely approximating a normal or Gaussian distribution. You may have encountered portrayal of population characteristics like this before. All this means is that a few people have very low resistance to stressors (left-hand tail), a few people have very high resistance (right-hand tail) and most of us are about average and are in the middle (under the hump).

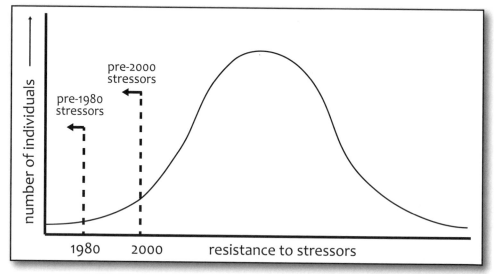

As we increase the level of stressors in our environment, we move from left to right. As we do this, we move into the hump area and we include more and more people who can't tolerate the stressors. The problem goes beyond pesticides, herbicides, fungicides, petrochemicals, engine and power plant effluents and the like; it extends into the realm of infectious organisms and challenges to our immune systems. Overuse of antibiotics during the last several decades may be a major instigator for ASD. I also believe that vaccinations, too many at once or given when even minor illness is present, have been contributing factors. I believe this because I've witnessed, at meetings, thousands of parents indicating that there is a vaccination/time association with the onset of their children's ASD. Whether or not the vaccine itself is an issue is not something I'm professionally qualified to judge. But, the period of inflammation that may follow a vaccination is something that concerns me, and inflammation in ASD is something I've studied. Persistent inflammation promotes the autistic condition, and it's perhaps the biggest obstacle to relieving many autistic traits.

Poor nutrition and an indoor lifestyle that lacks exercise, fresh air and sunshine also are influencing factors, both for pregnant moms and for infants. You either eat healthy foods or you take nutritional supplements, and for some of us, good health requires both. You hear on TV that "sugar is sugar is sugar"! I hope you don't believe that. If you do, then when you learn about digestive enzymes and the special carbohydrate diet, you will find another complication in our world. And hey, either you get sunshine regularly or you take vitamin D_3, or your health will suffer. Don't expect genes alone to determine health or longevity – especially not in our polluted world.

There is also the spectrum of autisms/ASD which contributes significantly to the increased incidence. Honestly, there are a whole lot of strangely-behaved children and young adults who are now called autistic. Their behaviors usually include some autistic or "autistic-like" traits. Decades ago they weren't given the diagnosis of autism, and most importantly, there were far fewer of them. I view the creation of the spectrum as an expansion of the diagnosis made necessary by the ever-increaing types and amounts of acquired stressors.

Referring back to the bell-shaped curve shown above, we don't have to continue "progressing" to the right – the direction of increased inflammation-causing stressors. But, as a society, we don't seem to know how to stop this progression, and worse, many don't even recognize that we are doing this.

ASD – A Persistent Maladaptive Condition

By my tally, over fifty different toxic and infectious insults have been accused of causing autism. While many of these might be triggers for some form of ASD, the commonality is oxidant stress, probably oxidant damage to cells or tissue, and a period of inflammatory response, during which body makes adjustments to metabolism, immunologic defense, and sometimes to mental function. It's persistent inflammation that locks in much of ASD. The inflammation is persistent because the body's defense mechanisms for cleaning house (detoxication) or identifying and eliminating alien microorganisms (immune response) aren't up to today's challenges.

The various stressors that instigate and/or perpetuate an autistic condition can be different, sequential and cumulative. If the messengers of inflammation (cytokines) go up and don't come down, that's very bad for autism. It results in a maladaptive response that won't go away until the inflammation does. You should be aware that the topic of inflammation in autism still is controversial. Considering only the intestinal tract, I have read clinical reports and heard doctors lecture numerous times, and there is little consensus or agreement. Many (not all) gastroenterologists find digestive enzyme deficiencies but deny the presence of significant dysbiosis, and they are divided about inflammation. Many immunologists (not all) report elevations of inflammatory markers (cytokines), but maldigestion just isn't their forte, though some do acknowledge food reactivities. Doctors who have gone looking for dysbiotic gut flora have found plenty. The lab tests I've seen, the parent testimonies, and the balance of presented and published studies have put me in the inflammation camp. I believe it - not for all but for a majority.

The Overall Objectives

So, what are the goals for nutritional intervention? Well, it's pretty simple to say but not so simple to do. The first step is to stop or at least reduce the tissue distress and inflammation. If you look at ARI Pub 34 (see Appendix), you will see that special diets, digestive enzymes and antioxidant/anti-inflammatory supplements including melatonin are helpful for 60-70% in terms of improved behaviors (n>20,000 – that's over 20,000 parent reports.)

While we concentrate on normalizing intestinal functions, we can also use a few nutritional aids to reduce the brain inflammation of ASD, such as giving melatonin and taurine. I don't know how many ASD victims have brain inflammation, or at least activated glial cells in the brain, but indications are it's a lot. (Vargas et al. Ann Neurol 81, 2005, 67-81).

Then there are some other major intervention goals that we should strive for – (1) enhancing cellular energy delivery, (2) improving energy utilization, and (3) improving neuronal synchrony. While there can be complicated pathologies behind deficient cellular energy and neuronal asynchrony, there are some easy-to-use nutritional aids that may be helpful.

So, to help the ASD person in our care, our work assignment is –
- Reduce oxidant stress and inflammation in intestine and brain
- Bolster detoxication – get the toxicants out – which contributes to lowering inflammation
- Re-regulate and properly focus immune response
- Enhance energy delivery and utilization, brain and body
- Improve neuronal synchrony and communication among neuronal networks.

All of these are objectives that nutritional supplements can help you achieve. But they can't do any of these jobs alone. Digestive enzymes can do a lot to reduce intestinal inflammation, but they aren't a substitute for excluding trouble-making foods from the diet. Oral glutathione really does help to detoxify and remove many toxicants from the body, but it's unlikely to overcome the body's toxic load if you live near a toxic dump site or next to a farm that has the insecticide dicofol sprayed around. An immune system will never work right if there is mercury roaming around in body tissues. Cell mitochondria are stressed when they have to remove excessive organic acids and transport certain antibiotic medications, as well as produce energy. All of these tasks require L-carnitine and its transporters. When these needs compete, cellular energy production is going to lose out. To make matters worse, carnitine is made in the body by a process that's hampered in many autistics – methylation. There's more about this process in the Glossary.

Neuronal synchrony won't happen until oxidant stress, energy delivery and methylation are significantly improved. Neuronal synchrony is what you want first, because it leads to mental perception, comprehension, and expressive speech. But biologically, in autism, you can't have it first. First, you're going to have to alleviate the maladaptive response condition that holds ASD in place.

In summary, don't expect much expressive speech right away and don't expect it to come with nutritional intervention alone. There's a lot more that's required.

BACKGROUND & PREREQUISITE STRATEGIES

Let's focus on some prerequisite strategies that allow nutritional intervention to succeed. In most cases, if you don't do these, you'll only be wasting money on bottles of supplements. More importantly, you'll be wasting valuable time. The earlier in life that we can intervene with these strategies, the more likely we are to improve the condition.

~ Prerequisite Strategy 1 ~

Remove/avoid potentially toxic stressors – chemical stuff that can cause detoxication challenges and inflammation

These are substances that are likely to make autistic traits worse and that may be the very stressors that brought on the problem in the first place. I wish we knew what all of them are – I surely don't. But I do have a list of prime suspects that include pesticides, herbicides and fungicides, especially the organochlorine and organophosphate types. Why? A short history lesson will tell you why.

Organochlorine Toxicants – The Beginning of Acquired ASD

In the 1930s, many research chemists were busy adding chlorine atoms to organic chemical molecules such as benzene. Chemists use the word "organic" to mean a substance composed mostly of carbon atoms and often containing oxygen and hydrogen atoms as well. Organic chemicals can be of natural origin, such as the hydrocarbons (hydrogen plus carbon atoms) in crude oil, or they can be man-made and may only be found in places we'd call polluted. Benzene does exist naturally (in crude oil), but virtually all of it that we work with today is manufactured from other natural chemicals in crude oil. (Note: "natural" doesn't necessarily mean good or healthy! Neither does "organic"!)

Some objectives of adding chlorine to organics included development of antiseptics, insecticides and fungicides, solvents for oils and waxes, and chemicals to aid fabric dyeing and finishing. Synthesis of dichlorobenzyl alcohol was patented in 1932, and it was used as an antiseptic as was chlorinated cresol. (Cresol is a fancied-up form of benzene that's less volatile but just as toxic.)

Chlorinated naphthalene, a solvent for fats and oils and a laboratory chemical, came into use during 1933-36. Chlorophenol, an antiseptic, was described in the Journal of the American Chemical Society in 1935, and preparation of trichlorophenol, a bacteriocide, fungicide and preservative was published in 1931. It was later used in the Russian chemical process industry. So, humans placed organochlorines in the biosphere in the 1930s, and usage patterns indicate that we weren't very careful about how they got used or where they went.

In 1939, chemist Paul Müller, working for Geigy AG (Switzerland), "rediscovered" a potent insecticide while pursuing Geigy's quest for a poison for moths and carpet beetles. Assembled from two molecules of chlorobenzene and one molecule of chloral (trichloroacetaldehyde), he made dichlorodiphenyltrichloroethane, which obviously needed an abbreviation, "DDT". The compound had been synthesized and described long before, but it hadn't been put to any commercial use. During 1940 and 1941, demonstrations of DDT's usefulness occurred, including in the US. Full-scale industrial production occurred in 1942. In 1943, the Allies used it in Naples to suppress a typhus epidemic by applying it directly to soldiers and civilians to kill body lice. The disease is also carried by fleas and ticks, and they're killed by DDT, too.

In 1943 Dr Leo Kanner, Director of the Child Psychiatry Clinic at Johns Hopkins Hospital, published the first psychiatric description of autism ("Autistic Disturbances of Affective Contact"). Hans Asperger described the syndrome bearing his name in 1944. By 1948, DDT was in worldwide use, and Paul Müller was awarded a Nobel Prize. By the end of the 1950s, DDT and other chlorinated cyclic organics (cyclodienes, benzenes and cyclohexanes) had wide use in agriculture, forestry, manufacture of building materials and pest control. But adverse effects on people and animals, especially birds and fish, began to be noticed, and "toxicity" gained emphasis in the industrial chemists' lexicon. Rachel Carson authored Silent Spring in 1962. In 1972, use of DDT in the US was restricted to the military, to medical use (by prescription), and to public health emergencies.

Meanwhile, the agricultural and chemical process industries were busy inventing and commercializing replacement and alternative products. The list is long. Lindane was one; it got booted out of the US in 1977 (but it's still imported for medical use against lice and scabies). Per Sittig's reference text, Pesticides and Agricultural Chemicals (2005), some of the organochlorines in recent use include: alachlor, chlorothalonil, chlorphyrifos (an organochloro-phosphorothiolate), dicofol, endosulfan, trichlorfon.

Dicofol is an analog of DDT and is manufactured from it. Dicofol is dichlordiphenyltrichloro-ethanol (ethanol instead of DDT's ethane). Dicofol has one oxygen atom on its molecule that DDT does not have; that's the only difference. Dicofol has preparation and use patents dating from 1957; major agricultural use came in the 1970s. There are at least 18 different trade names for it, and legally-allowable dicofol residues are stated for 50 food crops (40 CFR, 180.163).

Endosulfan is another organochlorine; it has a descriptive chemical name that's too long to recite. It was patented in 1961 and has been produced in the US by four chemical companies. There are 25 other manufacturers worldwide. Maximum allowable residue levels for endosulfan are stated for over 70 US food crops and for over a dozen other agricultural items including animal byproducts, hulls, straw and cotton (40 CFR 180.182). Recently, there's good news for us on endosulfan. Announced in May 2011 is a global treaty banning use worldwide (Chem & Engng News, May 9, p 15).

Mechanisms of dicofol and endosulfan toxicities are described in <u>Casarett & Doull's Toxicology</u>, McGraw-Hill, 5th Ed. (1996) 649-654. Both the DDT-type (dicofol) and the endosulfan-type inhibit neuronal energy, chemistry and electrical charge activity. Both insecticides are fully capable of causing loss of neuronal synchrony and loss of neuron-to-neuron communication.

Okay, so far, there's a time correlation and a theoretical toxicology connection between ASD and certain organochlorines. That doesn't prove causation. But then, along came Dr. Eric Roberts from the Public Health Institute in Oakland, CA, along with helpers from the California Department of Health Services and the School of Public Health, University of California, Berkeley. Roberts et al. studied the incidence of autism in the California Central Valley and correlated that incidence with maternal residence near sites of pesticide application. They tested 249 different hypotheses, including those related to dozens of different agricultural chemicals and exposure parameters. Four of these met statistically significant criteria for causal relevance, and all four involved application of organochlorine pesticides, specifically dicofol and endosulfan (Environ. Health Perspect <u>115</u> no.10, Oct. 2007 1482-1489). **Per the Roberts et al study, incidence of autism exactly correlated with time of exposure, distance from the area of application, and with the poundage of organochlorines that were used.**

As sure as smoking is a cause of lung cancer, these organochlorines are one cause of autism. We have relevant neurotoxicity, we have dose-response, plus a chronological match, a geographical match, and a chemical stressor history that goes back to the time of Drs. Kanner and Asperger. That's about as close as science can get to proof of cause – unless we purposely expose pregnant moms to this junk. Let's not!

I have provided a list of agricultural chemicals to specifically avoid in the Appendix, with the understanding that it was compiled to the best of my knowledge and is most definitely imperfect and incomplete. If you are aware of the presence or use of any of these chemicals and you are pregnant or with your ASD loved one, run, don't walk, in the other direction.

Organophosphate Toxicants

Another group of harmful chemicals invented by man and commercialized during the second half of the 20th century is the organophosphates. Although mostly used as pesticides and herbicides, some of the most toxic chemicals on earth are organophosphates - the ones used as nerve gases: "tabun" (GA), "sarin" (GB), "soman" (GD), and VX. Organophosphates or "OP"s as they now are nicknamed, were first synthesized in the late 1930s in Germany (Farbenfabriken Bayer AG). Fortunately, these chemicals were not used militarily during World War II. Only one government ever used an OP nerve gas intentionally: Iraq used sarin against Kurdish settlements in northern Iraq in 1988. The United States was among the military powers that manufactured and stockpiled OP nerve gases. The problem we've been contending with during the last decade is safe disposal of them.

OPs inhibit cholinesterase. Cholinesterase is an enzyme that's present throughout the body and that destroys excess acetylcholine (produced in nerve tissue). Acetylcholine stimulates muscle contraction while cholinesterase acts at the nerve-muscle junction to prevent excessive or continued contraction. OPs knock out cholinesterase, allowing uncontrolled nerve-muscle stimulation by acetylcholine. This toxic action by OPs can adversely affect the central, sympathetic and parasympathetic nervous systems.

During the First Gulf War (1991), US military troops attacked a munitions storage area at Khamisiya, Iraq, and sarin and cyclosarin nerve gases were released. Some troops were acutely exposed while about 100,000 more were possibly exposed to low levels of these nerve agents (per Duke University Professor Abou-Donia, a recognized expert on this subject). Besides the acute effect of inhibiting cholinesterase, OP agents are reported to cause chronic problems including immune dysregulation, memory loss, muscle and joint pain, and gastrointestinal difficulties. Long-term psychopathologic-neurologic lesions resulting from OP insecticide exposure are well described in Casarett & Doull's Toxicology, 5th Ed., 656-59.

According to Chemical and Engineering News (July 11, 2005), VX destruction in the US was temporarily halted in 2005 following (a) a 30-gallon spill and (b) realization that a very flammable byproduct was being produced by the neutralization process. The procedure involved shipping VX from Newport, Indiana to the DuPont Company in New Jersey for neutralization followed by disposal in the Delaware River. At last report (2005), 3000 gallons of VX had been neutralized, leaving about 250,000 gallons still to be treated/disposed of. I do not know the current status of VX or other OP warfare stockpiles, but I hope we've gotten rid of them properly. While we'd like to think that the US populace has been protected from exposure to OP warfare agents, the published record, limited as it is, does not inspire confidence. Neither does the fact that the state of New Jersey has the highest per capita incidence of autism in the US.

An unresolved question is whether OPs cause gene damage that can be passed on to the next human generation (i.e., epigenetic damage). You'd think we'd be wise enough to find that out before we spray them around, wouldn't you!

Are OPs connected clinically to autism or ASD? Definitely yes. The biochemical links are complicated and reside deep in the metabolic pathway that leads from the nutritionally essential amino acid methionine to homocysteine and on to cysteine and glutathione. Along that molecular journey there's a pitfall, one that homocysteine can fall into. Once it's in the pit, it either gets rescued or it cannot move on toward cysteine and glutathione formation. There is an enzyme that rescues homocysteine from the pitfall. That enzyme was virtually unknown to science until OPs came along and researchers decided to learn how the body detoxifies some of them. They found an enzyme that would do the job of dismantling some OPs and named it "paraoxonase" or PON for short. Guess what – PON is the enzyme that rescues homocysteine from the pitfall - getting stuck as homocysteine thiolactone. But is this human enzyme supposed to be burdened with OP cleanup duty? Of course not. Here's the citation for the clinical study directly linking autism in North America with certain OPs: D'Amelio M, Ricci I, et al. "Paraoxonase gene variants are associated with autism in North America, but not in Italy: possible regional specificity in gene-environment interactions" Mol Psychiatry 2005 Nov;10(11):1006-16.

Other Toxicants of Concern

Other implicated chemicals include some drugs including the notorious thalidomide ones used a few decades ago, and valproate or valproic acid, used today to control some types of seizures. Valproate, by the way, is partly cleared from cells by L-carnitine, a natural body substance and a nutritional quantity that often is needed by those with ASD (see section on L-carnitine in this book, in the section, Nutrient Descriptions and Use Information).

There's another commonly-used medicine that I advise you to be wary of – acetaminophen. (It's called paracetamol in the UK.) The primary metabolism (detoxication) route the body uses to get rid of acetaminophen is to sulfate it. But sulfation is hindered in many with ASD, as reported by Dr. Rosemary Waring and others. Failing that, the body cleans up acetaminophen (or its oxidized daughter product) with glutathione – something else that's often in short supply in ASD per about a dozen clinical studies. Dr. Peter Good has published a thought-provoking article on acetaminophen and autism, and I recommend it to you (*Alternative Medicine Review* 14 no.4 (2009) 364-72).

Then there's a group of industrially-made chemicals that have been and are being outlawed but that are very persistent in the environment. These are biphenyls to which chlorine or its chemical cousin bromine has been added. Phenyl is very similar to benzene and a biphenyl is a molecule that includes two phenyls linked together. "PCB"s are polychlorinated biphenyls; they have been used as lubricant additives, hydraulic fluids, electrical power transformer fluid, pesticide extenders, etc. PBBs and PBDEs ("penta") are polybrominated biphenyls and polybrominated diphenyl chemicals. Mostly, these are (were) flame retardants. Not to be outdone by its sister chemical bromine, chlorine shows up in fire retardants, too. "Tris" or chlorinated tris is still in some baby products despite being outlawed for baby clothes decades ago – beware of baby carriers and car seats made with polyurethane foam. That stuff may contain tris (TDCPP or penta DBE). Unfortunately, you're not likely to know when this junk is around. Besides textiles, it's in lake and river sediments, dumps, soils, and in areas of prior use that may no longer be recognized as such.

Next, there are certain elements (minerals) that are possibly causative, or at least have some complicity, for ASD – mercury (Hg), lead (Pb), antimony (Sb), and arsenic (As). These elements have been implicated because in some clinical studies, they have been measured to be excessive in individuals with ASD, relative to lab reference ranges or relative to control populations.

ASD patient history indicates exposure at levels consistent with expected toxicity – as with mercury in Thimerosal in vaccine fluids prior to 2005.

The symptoms of toxicity and the biochemical effects match those of some autistic traits.

There is a geographical match between environmental contamination and ASD incidence – as with mercury in Texas and antimony in New Jersey.

However, I see several serious problems with placing a lot of blame for autism on these potentially toxic elements. Granted, they certainly can aggravate the situation by adding to the total toxic load. But unlike the organochlorines and organophosphates, we don't have time-matching with the beginnings of autism or with increase in ASD incidence to its now-epidemic level. During the 1850s-70s, mercury was dumped all over the central California watershed by gold mining/refining operations. Where is the history of autism? Ore smelters that release these toxic elements were operating for decades before the incidence of autism became alarming. We took the mercury out of latex paints 30 years ago and also the tetraethyl lead out of gasoline and the lead pigments out of paints and the incidence of autism went up in the 1980s, 1990s, and past 2000, not down. A few years ago, we took Thimerosal out of almost all the vaccines, and saw only a minor respite in the ASD incidence.

During the following years, the incidence resumed its ascent and now, with less mercury and less lead being added to our biosphere, we have the ASD incidence up to about one per 100 births (100 per 10,000 instead of the 5 per 10,000 of 40 years ago).

There is recent news of possible genomic damage from mercury contamination of grandparents resulting in increased incidence of autism in grandchildren (*Autism Research Review International* vol 25, no.3, page 1, ARI 2011). In my opinion, this research merits attention and support; our present sins and the sins of the past are contributing to the spectrum of autism that we have now.

It is a good idea to avoid these potential toxicants and to have them removed from the body (detoxification therapy) if your doctor believes they are present at excessive levels. But that's not something you do early on per my experience. Instead, you clean up the environment that you're exposed to (or exit the dirty environment), and you bolster nutritional status. Delay the detoxification treatments until they are better tolerated. When is that? Well, that's something your doctor has to figure out.

Purifying Your Living Space, Food and Drink

• Buy healthy foods from reliably pure sources – organic foods if you can afford them. The Environmental Working Group publishes an annual list of "The Dirty Dozen": the foods with the most pesticide residues. Use of the list may help you prioritize when to go organic. www.organic.org. For 2011, these were: peaches, apples, sweet bell peppers, celery, nectarines, strawberries, cherries, pears, grapes (imported), spinach, lettuce, potatoes.

• Use pure water – have yours tested. Some tap water is better than some bottled water. Glass bottled water (hard to find) usually eliminates plasticizer chemicals (incl. phthalates). Beware of water-borne molds, and organic chemicals such as the chlorinated and brominated ones. Special testing is required to quantitate most of these contaminants.

• In 1995, the Environmental Health Center-Dallas (William Rea, MD, Director) studied various spring water sources and published a list of good-quality ones (W.J. Rea, Chemical Sensitivity, vol.4 page 2364-65, Lewis Publishers, 1997. Some good ones include:

   • Mountain Valley, (spring water) Hot Springs, AK
   • Calistoga (spring), Calistoga, CA
   • Golden Nectar (well water), UT
   • Deep Rock (artesian) Denver CO
   • LaCroix (deep well) LaCrosse WI
   • Saratoga (artesian), Saratoga NY
   • Poland (spring) S. Poland ME

• Location – check whether you're near a toxic dump site, downwind from a chemical plant, petroleum refinery, or a coal-fired power plant. If you can afford to move, then do so. If you can't then look after food and water quality and get some air purifiers for the rooms in your home. This won't eliminate excessive toxicant exposure, but it will help a bunch.

• Clean up the living areas and get rid of any stored pesticide, herbicide, fungicide, or other toxicant-containing sprays, bottles or cans. Use these outside, if you must, and only when the ASD individual is absent from the premises – don't keep them around. And you don't have to use chemicals for pest control – see George Ware, Complete Guide to Pest Control with and without Chemicals, Thomsen Publications, Fresno CA (1988) or go online and look for information on environmentally safe and human-safe pest control procedures. Ditto for lawn and garden care.

- Got new textiles (rugs, carpets, drapes, etc)? Cotton and wool are the best, while nylon and plastic (polypropylene) are the worst. Rayon and acetate outgas less than the other synthetics and are usually okay. Watch out for pad materials and adhesives; these can cause problems. On floors, natural wood (nailed/screwed) and ceramic tile that is cemented or grouted (not glued) are best. Vinyl tiles, self-stick tiles and linoleum will outgas chemical vapors. I advise avoiding these.

- You will need to look at all of the products you use in your home, because so many things are likely to become a problem for your child. Exile cigarette smokers to the outside of your home. Many cleaning products, especially anything that comes in a spray can, should not be used. Perfumed soap, shampoo, laundry detergent, deodorant, aftershave, hair spray, cosmetics – the list goes on. Try to get unscented versions of the ones you can't stop using. Hypoallergenic products are preferred; most of these are unscented. Forget fabric softeners. There are "green" websites that will give you alternative cleaning strategies – baking-soda-and-water paste makes a very acceptable oven cleaner, for example. You may find that going through this process will help other family members as well. Assuming that your autistic family member is biologically related to the rest of you, it's very possible that the whole family has somewhat reduced detox capability.

Maureen McDonnell, R.N., a long-time student and researcher in the autism field, has a very useful website that can help you with some of these issues: www.SOKHOP.com.

~ Prerequisite Strategy 2 ~

Remove/Avoid Infectious Stressors – microorganisms and their toxins that can lead to inflammation; cease excessive use of antibiotic medications

A big part of ASD has to do with dysregulated responses to immune system challenges that go on and on, or that occur sequentially with differing microorganisms/toxins. These acquired stressors may have been present during the gestation period, during infancy or perhaps in early childhood. And what's identified as an infectious agent in a 5 year old with ASD may or may not have been the primary causative culprit. Infections that are not expediently overcome lead to inflammation, which becomes a persistent signal to certain genes that they should change expression and come to the rescue with new battle plans – plans that don't work in ASD.

When cells responsible for defense attack the body's own tissue instead, we call it an autoimmune response or disease – a type of dysregulation in which self is not clearly distinguished from foreign material. The chances of this happening are vastly increased when there is persistent inflammation and constant activation of immune cell defenses. There now are many published clinical studies reporting immune dysregulation and autoimmune responses as part of the pathology of autism. A lot of these are due to acquired infectious stressors that we've got to eliminate if we want nutritional therapy to have significant benefit.

Let's start our infectious stressor avoidance strategy by reviewing some microorganisms that I believe to cause symptoms of ASD in some individuals.

Yeast overgrowth – a historical case

Most gastroenterologists who have examined autistic children will tell you, as they've told me, "intestinal yeast is not a problem for autistics". Well, maybe that's because they don't practice in the San Francisco Bay Area, Southern Louisiana, or around the Gulf Coast. As with all scientific proofs, all I need to refute this misconception is one documented case, and that's the case of Duffy Mayo. It was described at length in the *Los Angeles Times*, Section VIII, Sunday Sept. 25, 1983. Five year-old Duffy lived in San Francisco and had twice been diagnosed by psychiatrists as autistic. It wasn't until Alan Levin, MD, a San Francisco allergist and immunologist, examined Duffy that the specific diagnosis of severe intestinal candidiasis was made. The Mayos stripped their house of moldy stuff, all of the carpeting went to the dump, and Dr. Levin put Duffy on nystatin to combat the candida excess. Things improved markedly when the family visited Italy, an area of drier climate. But Duffy relapsed upon return to San Francisco. Then, the Mayos moved to drier, nearby Walnut Creek and upped Duffy's nystatin medication. Soon his autistic symptoms disappeared, he began reading and making progress with speech therapy. At the time the newspaper article was written, Duffy no longer had the diagnosis of autism.

Of course, Duffy didn't have "genetic" autism – he had internal drunkenness from alcohol and aldehydes produced by a huge intestinal yeast overgrowth ("auto-brewery syndrome"). But then, what is autism? It's a collection of behavioral traits including lack of communication skills that can be due to dozens of acquired toxicant or infectious stressors – with or without many possible genetic faults, some of which are severe while others would never be a problem absent the stressors. Forty percent of PKU (phenylketoniuria) infants developed autistic traits before we knew what to do for PKU (Scandinavian data per Karl Reichelt, MD). Now we know what PKU is, and that it is a specific diagnosis. But this is what we're up against – a disorder with lots of possible causes ranging from almost purely acquired problems like severe intestinal yeast overgrowth, to almost purely genetic factors like PKU.

Bacterial dysbiosis and excessive use of antibiotic medications

During the 1970s, a group of British researchers at the United Kingdom Food Research Institute (Norwich) decided to study clostridia (genus clostridium), a group of anerobic, spore-forming bacteria. Many of these are causative for serious diseases. Anerobic means they thrive in the absence of air, and spore-forming means that when threatened, they morph into a protected, refractory oval-shaped dormancy to wait out the threat. The last time I counted, there were about two dozen species of clostridia including ones that cause botulism, gangrene, tetanus, and intestinal distress – colitis and diarrhea (Clostridium difficile).

The British researchers, led by Dr. Sidney Elsden, published three papers on what clostridia produce when they feed on amino acids, as might occur with maldigestion and malabsorption. The particular bug we're interested in here is C. difficile. When it feeds on phenylalanine, tyrosine or tryptophan, it produces phenylpropionic acid (PPA) among other chemicals. If that is absorbed into the bloodstream, the liver can detoxify this chemical by "hydroxylation" to HPPA, or DHPPA (doubly hydroxylated). Some other clostridia (C. sporogenes, C. botulinum) produce HPPA directly. C. difficile also produces indoleacetic acid and the "fancy" benzene I mentioned earlier in the DDT narrative - cresol, para-cresol to be exact. Para-cresol is very poisonous. Most of the clostridia bugs also produce various short-chain fatty acids, including propionic acid. This occurs when they ingest four other dietary amino acids that are essential for humans – valine, leucine, isoleucine and threonine. Sorry for all the chemistry here, but it's important if only for word recognition of what has been discovered in ASD individuals.

At the 1996 Autism Society of America (ASA) national conference, Dr. William Shaw reported analytical identification of hydroxylated PPA in the urine of autistics. He attributed it, correctly in my opinion, to bacterial dysbiosis. In 2002, Anderson and Bendell reported analytical identification of a metabolite of tryptophan, "IAG", in the urine of autistics – *J. of Pharmacy & Pharmacology,* 54(2), 2002, 295-98. IAG can come from indole-acetic acid that various clostridia make from tryptophan. Using an animal model (rats), Dr. Derrick MacFabe and his colleagues at Western Ontario University have demonstrated autistic behaviors following exposures to propionic acid, PA – *Behav. Brain Res.* 176 (1) 2007, 149-69; Neuropharmacol 54 (6) 2008, 901-11. What all this means is that some ASD individuals present various chemical markers showing the presence of clostridia. One of the markers is related to a short-chain organic acid (propionic acid) that, in rats, produces autistic-like traits. Also, realize that propionic acid is something that L-carnitine is supposed to remove from cell mitochondria.

All of this would be just another "red herring" for ASD except for three things. First, many of our ASD children have maldigestion, malabsorption and colitis. Second, if treated successfully for intestinal clostridial dysbiosis, the DHPPA/IAG markers decrease or normalize, colitis ceases, inflammation markers decrease and behavioral improvement often follows. Third, a daughter metabolite of propionic acid, methylmalonic acid, "MMA" is reported by doctors to be above normal levels (lab reference ranges) for about 25% of untreated children with ASD.

So, why don't we just give antibiotic medications to kill these bad bugs in the gut? Up until a few years ago, that seemed to work. That's what some doctors did for ASD when there was evidence of dysbiosis, and it's what many general practitioners continue to do routinely for bacterial infections or as a preventative measure when infection is a concern. In the 2005 book, Autism: Effective Biomedical Treatments, authored by Dr. Sidney Baker and me, I mentioned use of Vancomycin (plus probiotics!) for intestinal dysbiosis. That's because doctors treating ASD told me it worked. As of 2010, I'm hearing a completely different story – maybe because the additional probiotic requirement wasn't met or maybe because C. difficile is smarter (more adaptable) than we thought.

I'm sorry to have to tell you that continued use of such antibiotics (vancomycin, amoxicillin, flagyl, ciprofloxacin, all the fluoroquinolones antibiotics, and the cephalosporins too) has led to a big problem – antibiotic-resistant gut bugs including a particularly nasty and hard-to-kill version of C. difficile.

There's a bit more to the antibiotic story that you need to know. Cephalosporin is a genus of soil-inhabiting fungi with the ability to kill invading and nearby bacteria. Beginning in the late 1940s, there was a search for something that could eradicate bacteria that had become penicillin resistant. Such an antibiotic was found in a strain of cephalosporin growing near a sewage outlet on the island of Sardinia. During the 1950s and 60s, various agents extracted from cephalosporins were patented and commercial synthesis procedures were designed to manufacture these agents.

Cephalosporins work by producing chemicals that are transported into the cell wall of the bacterium, which they cause to be unstable and susceptible to penetration by ions, salts, and other substances that disrupt the bacterium's ability to grow. Three generations of cephalosporins have been commercialized and they often are prescribed today for various bacterial infections.

There are two problems with cephalosporins –

1. They can change the normal flora content of the colon and allow overgrowth of Clostrida, including C. difficile (Facts & Comparisons, Jan 2000, page 1242).
2. They depend upon carnitine transport mechanisms for their movement, including removal from our cells. Removal of certain other types of antibiotics also depends on carnitine transporters, and so do propionates, valproate and short-chain organic acids. (See later section on L-carnitine.) I am told informally by researchers that burdening the carnitine transporter system with synthetic/foreign chemicals may, in some cases, result in clogging up the works. Those infants and children with predisposition to carnitine dysregulation/deficiency or to mitochondrial dysfunction would do well to avoid cephalosporin antibiotics. Unfortunately, with today's knowledge and procedures, we have no idea who these infants/children are. So my advice to you – avoid the cephalosporins, too.

To summarize, some with ASD have intestinal distress that includes maldigestion and malabsorption. These conditions can lead to the growth of bad bugs in the gut. The bugs are bad because they produce toxic stuff, some of which gets absorbed into the bloodstream. Clinicians have found these toxins in ASD individuals by doing lab tests. Animal model research shows at least one such substance produces the symptoms of autism. During the last five years, immunology and pharmacology researchers have found that many antibiotics cause or worsen intestinal dysbiosis of the type we find in some with ASD. So, what are we to do?

Killing persistent pathogens naturally

I did another study, this time on herbal remedies for Clostridia and other pathogenic gut flora. I wish to emphasize that C. difficile is only one of many suspects in the group of potentially harmful germs that researchers are isolating and identifying in their studies of ASD. I do wish these researchers would stand up soon and start hollering about what they've found. There's more to this story.

Why herbals? I was struck by the revelation that plant antibiotic systems involve more than one chemical agent. There's the antibiotic and then there's at least one other chemical weapon which disables the target microbe's defense mechanism. The problem with single antibiotic agents is that some microbes can "pump" the agent back out again – before it has time to work. Wounding some germs instead of killing them might allow them to adapt either by changing cell chemistry, or by morphing into a protected, dormant form (spores). The barberry bush can kill staph aureus quite efficiently with a one-two punch of antibiotic (berberine) plus a chemical agent that jams the staph's defense (5'-methoxyhydnocarpin).

Do our pharmaceutical antibiotics work like this? No, they don't. And that's why we're having to constantly invent new ones.

What works are certain herbals (complete ones, not extracts) or oils from herbals such as thyme and oregano that knock out clostridia, bacillus, citrobacter, klebsiella, proteus, salmonella, and staphylococcus. Turmeric (curcumin) is a great antioxidant and anti-inflammatory to be used while thyme and oregano are doing their killing work. A hired-gun microorganism that is a yeast, Saccharomyces boulardii, also can be very helpful. S. boulardii is a "probiotic" (good bug) that gets rid of unwanted yeasts/fungi, and that helps eradicate clostridia. Other probiotics that help, but can't do the job alone, are Lactobacillus plantarum and Lactobacillus rhamnosis. Use these herbal and probiotic agents to help achieve a healthy population of intestinal flora in individuals with ASD. If there's a relapse, use them again, or better, use maintenance levels continually. See your ASD-experienced physician or nutritionist for amounts, or follow the supplement manufacturer's recommendations. Look for capsule versions of the herbs.

~ Prerequisite Strategy 3 ~

Fix the Diet

During the last thirty years while I worked to help those with autism and to counsel parents about remedial options, I encountered two significant misconceptions. One is the ridiculous position of medical authorities that behavior is not influenced by diet. The second – just as ridiculous – is the idea that with the right nutritional supplements you don't have to worry about diet.

The position of medical orthodoxy on diet and behavior is changing, finally! Evidence of this can be found at the American Academy of Pediatrics, in the "AAP Ground Rounds" article by Allison Schonwald, "ADHD and Food Additives Revisited", 2008, and in the journal editor's notes – "Thus, the overall findings of the study are clear and require that even we skeptics, who have long doubted parental claims of the effects of various foods on the behavior of their children, admit we might have been wrong."

I suspect, however, that it will still be a long time before this realization is applied to ASD. This, despite the published clinical/dietary studies of Reichelt, Knivsberg, Whitely, Shattock, Trajkovski and many others; despite the statistical compilation of parent experiences by Rimland; and despite the splendid efforts of Lisa Lewis, Karen Seroussi and others to popularize their findings on dietary interventions.

In my opinion, diet is a really big deal for many with ASD –especially the children. The foods that an ASD child eats can influence his/her condition in three ways.

1. He/she may be allergic to certain foods and eating such foods can provoke an inflammatory response – obviously, bad news. Often, people regularly eat foods to which they have an allergy. A maladaptive response follows which masks the problem and can lead to addiction to such foods. When the person stops eating the addictive food, he/she may have discomfort of some sort (headache) and feel a craving for the food. (Coffee is a common example in the adult world.) Usually, after a week, the craving is gone, the discomfort is gone, the person feels better than before, and is mentally sharp.

Not all allergy-producing foods do this. Many produce a prompt symptom such as a rash or stuffed-up nose; such foods are easily identified. The allergy-producing foods that we worry about most in ASD are the ones with subdued or delayed responses and that often do become addictive. Milk, other dairy products, and gluten-containing cereal grains are examples. What you may not realize is that there is a battle going on in the intestinal tract when these foods are regularly eaten by an addicted person.

2. Some foods are poorly digested and the partially digested bits can be biologically and neurologically active if absorbed into the body. Partially-digested parts of proteins are called peptides and some of these can act as neurotransmitters or as false signaling molecules for cells. These diet-source imposters can tell cells to do things that are quite inappropriate. With ASD we worry about peptides from casein (milk protein) and gluten (grain protein). Some milk peptides are "casomorphins", -morphin because they have morphine-like action on neurons – obviously addictive. A gluten peptide, gliadorphin (gluteomorphin) has the same effect.

   Of importance is the possibility of these peptides attaching to and inactivating tissue and cell proteins that are nearly identical to the intestinal protein (enzyme) that was supposed to digest them but didn't. This problem appears to be occurring for at least the subset of ASD individuals with elevated adenosine. That's about one in five autistic children, per the studies of Dr. Jill James. One of the enzymes that gets rid of excess adenosine is held in place by its binding protein, which is the same protein as the digestive enzyme dipeptidylpeptidase IV (DPP4). In the small intestine, DPP4 digests casomorphins, provided it's not inhibited by organophosphates, antibiotics or other stuff (e.g. mercury) that may grab onto it and clog up its workings. When adenosine goes up, inflammatory signaling can increase. Symptoms from this may take days to be evident while the individual may have a powerful craving for casein foods. DPP4, by the way, was isolated from human placental tissue by Dr. Püschel and others at the University of Kiel (Germany) with results published in 1982. In placental tissue, DPP4 has several purposes, one being a guardian protecting the fetus from harmful stuff. Per the study by Püschel, DPP4 is inactivated (wrecked) by organophosphate chemicals (insecticides) and by inorganic mercury (mercuric chloride). DPP4 is a very important protein in humans and we don't want it underperforming in ASD. Plant-source DPP4 analog is a digestive enzyme provided in several digestive-aid formulations for ASD and is highly recommended.

3. Foods that are not completely digested provide a feast for opportunistic flora that can live in the ASD individual's intestines. Poor digestion is a major cause of persistent intestinal dysbiosis. This occurs when digestive enzymes don't work right, and that's exactly what has been found with autism, as published by Drs. Horvath, Buie, Kushak and others. They document incomplete digestion of carbohydrates, complex sugars in particular. Their findings are consistent with the advisability of the "specific carbohydrate diet" ("SCD") for many ASD individuals. The SCD was developed by Elaine Gottschall; it avoids the sugars in

question, two of which are sucrose and isomaltose. The enzyme that digests them is the sucrase-isomaltase complex that lives in crypt and villous cells of the small intestine. Living in exactly the same place is their neighbor enzyme, DPP4. (See Gorvel et al, *Gastroenterology* <u>101</u> (3), 1991, p. 618-25.) Amazing coincidence!

The big problem with special diets is, which one? In most cases it's not possible to tell without trials. With this disease we do not learn much by averaging responses over an unsegregated sample of the ASD population. They're individuals. This also is one of the problems with medical orthodoxy's investigations of diet for ASD. Some do well on the specific carbohydrate diet (70%), some with a casein-free diet (55%), some with a gluten-free diet (about 50%), some with the low oxalate diet (50%), and some on the Feingold diet which avoids synthetics and artificial additives (60%). (I suggest that these additives be avoided by everyone, regardless of what other dietary strategies you might choose!)

Detailed procedures for meal-making and trying out a diet are beyond the scope of this book, but you will have to go through diet trials to give your child the best chance for success. A possible outcome is that a special diet has no discernable benefit. I think that holds for about one in four or five (20-25%) with ASD, and it holds more for older individuals than younger ones. Children with ASD tend to benefit more from diet therapy than do adults with ASD.

Here are some books that can help you work through the diet prerequisite to success.

Elaine Gottschall, <u>Breaking the Vicious Cycle: Intestinal Health Through Diet</u>. (Kirkton Press) August 1994.

Pamela Compart, MD and Dana Laake, <u>The Kid-Friendly ADHD & Autism Cookbook,</u> Fair Winds Press (Quayside Publishing), 2006

Julie Matthews, <u>Nourishing Hope</u> 2008; www.Healthful Living.com

Lisa Ackerman, "Journey Guide" 2007: TACA (Talk About Curing Autism), PO Box 12409, Newport Beach CA 92658, <u>www.tacanow.org</u>. See section 7, 'Dietary Intervention".

Lisa S. Lewis, Ph.D. and Karen Seroussi, see <u>Special Diets for Special Kids</u>, also the <u>Dietary Intervention Encyclopedia.</u> See the ANDI (Autism Network for Dietary Intervention) website, which has links in all directions to much useful information. <u>www.autismndi.com</u>.

Karen Seroussi, <u>Unraveling the Mystery of Autism and PDD – A Mother's Story of Research and Recovery</u>

Tips about Special Diets

Your job, perhaps coached by a doctor or nutritionist, will be to figure out if an exclusionary diet is beneficial, and if so, which one. The job involves trials of diets, trials that can take weeks or months to tell the tale. There is no nutritional or clinical test than can predict what foods to exclude or what diet to go to. There are some clues that you can uncover with testing, and I'll describe them. But the bottom line on diet is – try and see. When observed day to day, benefits from special diets can be gradual, almost imperceptible. But they can be tremendously beneficial over months of time. It helps to record your observations as you go.

With our son, we kept a daily food diary. We rotated foods by classification using a four day rotation diet. We excluded foods with artificial colors and flavors. We did take dairy foods out of his diet for a period of time; ditto with gluten foods. No matter what we did, he continued having unpredictable, violent, destructive tantrums, with stimming and all kinds of inappropriate behaviors. Finally, we did a food allergy test, and the IgG response to casein was off the chart high. Weeks after having no casein to eat, it was still off the chart high – I mean 10x higher than the "high number" at the right hand edge of the report sheet. After about six or seven weeks with no dietary casein he got a glass of milk. During the next 30 minutes, I got bitten; his mother got bitten (twice). Two windows were broken and furniture was damaged. Fortunately, his little sister, knowing the signs well, had locked herself in her bedroom.

Certainly not all children and adults with ASD will respond as ours did, but some will. I've heard similar stories from other parents. Sometimes it's a mistake on the diet or a cookie from Grandma or a milk chocolate that got sneaked in. And sometimes you'll just scratch your head and wonder why the eruption occurred.

Moms and dads, if you do an exclusionary diet with your ASD loved one and if you're unsure about its benefit, wait six or eight weeks and then provide a deliberate food challenge. When you do this, do NOT ever do it alone. You may need considerable physical help.

There are several actions you should take prior to diet trials. These are described elsewhere and I've listed them here in brief.

1. Remove toxicants from the environment or at least change the environment to the cleanest and purest degree that's possible.

2. Find a medical doctor, naturopath or (licensed) nutritional counselor who can order some basic clinical tests. Get this testing done before nutritional intervention. The health professional may have a series of tests that he/she uses for guidance. I recommend cooperation with their testing schedule – we all work best with familiar tools. I recommend at least the following tests initially.
    - Blood chemistry and CBC or basic metabolic profile
    - Thyroid status; iron status
    - Stool analysis with identification of bacteria, yeast and fungi and digestive markers
    - Hair element analysis (screening test), possibly followed by blood cell analysis and provoked urine analysis for essential and toxic elements if the hair report has suspicious results

3. With your health professional, get a detailed patient history with pertinent parent history as well.

4. The only nutritional intervention that I suggest starting before diet trials is use of digestive aids – that is, digestive enzymes. You will probably need digestive aid support no matter what diet is chosen and even if one isn't. There likely will be an initial week-to-ten-day period of worse-before-better with digestive enzymes – use activated charcoal to help control symptoms. (Please see the chapter on digestive enzymes.) If you really know what foods offend and what

diet will be of benefit, then it's okay to start the diet first and put the enzymes in after a few weeks – but you'll need to be correct about the diet. Actually, digestive enzymes are synergistic with the diet in bringing benefit.

The "Feingold diet" isn't an option – it's required along with trials of the other diets. The part about no junk food, no artificial food colors, flavors, etc. is absolutely necessary. The Candida diet (or low-sugar diet) in my opinion means you should serve foods with no added sugar. Limit the naturally high-sugar foods if the stool analysis shows yeast overgrowth. The stool analysis isn't foolproof, so your doctor may recommend trial doses of antifungal medications just to expose and knock off lurking yeast and fungi that don't show in the stool analysis. If the thyroid test shows a hypothyroid condition, then both the candida diet and the special carbohydrate diets are candidates. That's because there are likely to be increased amounts of sugar left in the intestinal tract (more on this in the Iodine section of the Minerals chapter).

The first requirement of any human diet is that it provides sufficient protein, carbohydrates, fats, and overall calories to meet nutritional needs for daily living, growth, repair of tissue, etc. Therefore, I strongly suggest that, if you are not knowledgeable about such matters, you become so, or find a nutritionist who can help you. Also, it is best to try the diets sequentially – that is, one after another.

I suggest starting with the casein-free diet for a 30 to 45 day period. If you're uncertain about benefit, do the food challenge with a glass of milk or a dish of ice cream, perhaps twice. Have help nearby. When you do the CF diet, you will probably need to supplement calcium; please see the Calcium section in the Minerals chapter.

After you've been using the CF diet for at least 30 days, you may start the gluten-free diet as an additional trial, or you can wait until you're sure about casein alone. I lean toward having a period during which both gluten and casein are avoided, because both are frequently problems for these kids. For the gluten-free diet, you often need 90 to 120 days to see benefits. Why all this time? The gut has to heal, inflammatory agents have to subside, absorbed toxicants and false neurotransmitters have to be metabolized out, and neuronal networks have to learn to say hello to one another.

You can test GF benefit usually after 60 days with a bowl of cream of wheat (flavored with salt, only). Again, have help nearby. When there's a reaction to a challenge meal, there will be a relapse in condition, but at least you'll know for sure that gluten foods are offenders, and you'll believe! (And any doubters in your family will too.) If there's no benefit to excluding gluten foods, then the GF diet isn't something you have to worry about.

The specific carbohydrate diet (SCD) scores 71% "got better" on ARI Publication 34, 2009. The diet excludes most foods containing disaccharides and polysaccharides (complex sugars). Subnormal disaccharidase enzyme activity is a problem in the small intestine of many with ASD. Most digestive enzyme formulations for autism and ASD now contain considerable disaccharidase potency, and this helps with carbohydrate tolerance and with the SCD.

If you've already started digestive enzyme use, then you've taken care of one potential problem related to high oxalates – use of lipase to digest dietary fat. In the intestine, fat ties up calcium; calcium then can't tie up oxalic acid, and it gets into the bloodstream. Only laboratory tests can tell you if this is happening and you'll need a doctor's order for such tests. When oxalate is high, try a low oxalate diet. You can give vitamin B_6 and restrict supplemental levels of glycine. Some are also helped by supplemental folic acid and taurine. Susan Owens has pioneered study of oxalate problems in autistic children and adults. She has shown that for some, a low-oxalate diet is beneficial. I suggest that you look this up on Google, using "Susan Owens AND low oxalate diet" as search terms. You will find a great deal of very helpful information.

Constipation, diarrhea, and intestinal distress all are signs that diet needs attention. Also, some laboratory tests can provide clues as to which diet may be beneficial.

- Ig levels to casein and gluten and other foods. These "allergy tests" are not foolproof and may have false positives
- Stool analysis with digestive markers and aerobic yeast/bacteria. Lots of yeast would be consistent with need for limiting certain carbohydrates (complex sugars). While it is very difficult to starve out yeast, there's no need to pamper them, either.
- Thyroid hormones. When they're low, increased amounts of unabsorbed carbohydrates, including sugars, may be left in the intestine.
- Urine oxalate levels – I recommend use of a hospital lab where prompt analysis of urine lessens the effect of ascorbate (vitamin C) becoming oxalate while the urine waits for analysis.

~ Prerequisite or Concurrent Strategy 4 ~

Relational Therapy and Special Ed Sessions

There is another part of the program that greatly increases your chances for success. Behaviors that are repeated, perhaps ritualistically, and often for no apparent reason, are called habits. Originally, most habits had a cause and there might have been positive or negative reinforcement with that cause. When I was a child, Mom taught me to bow-tie my shoelaces and then twist-knot the bows once more. Crawling around in the Illinois prairie, I'd lose a shoe if I didn't. And it was such a bother to tie them if they came undone while I was running around. I'm 71 now; I don't run around in prairies (they're long gone), but I still double-knot my shoe laces. Why? I tell myself it's so I don't have to bend down and retie laces, but the real reason is, it's a habit. Habits don't die so easily.

ASD has organic causes. It is not a behavior caused by unloving parents or by poor parenting. It is caused by defects in energy, connectivity and synchrony in the brain's neuronal networks, often coupled to distress and dysregulation of digestive, transport, and immune processes in the intestinal tissues. There is very close coordination between brain and gut in terms of neurotransmitters, signaling processes, and immune/defense functions. If we are skilled enough and lucky enough to intervene and improve the gut-brain disorder that exists in most with ASD, then we should be able to improve the set of behavioral and cognitive disorders that are called ASD.

To do that, we have to fade out the trained-in behaviors that are related to or are themselves autistic traits. Then we have to encourage learning skills that lead to new, appropriate behaviors and relationships with others. This won't happen automatically just because inflammation, immunity and metabolism are improved. Why should a person ask for something that has always been provided before? Why shouldn't he/she throw a tantrum to get what they want? It worked last time. It reduces the frustration level for everybody if the child can learn to make specific requests for what he or she wants or needs. Repaired biochemistry or not, you're going to need some expert help on behavior and learning.

Moms and dads, it's going to be hard for you to tell if you're making progress with nutritional therapy if you don't guide and test behavior and learning as you go along. Activities including play therapy, speech therapy, auditory integration, applied behavioral analysis, etc. will do wonders to bring out perception and response that biomedical treatments, including nutritional therapy, can make possible. And, if your orientation on this is opposite from mine – fine. Nutritional therapy can improve the new world that relational therapy opens up for your child. The fact is, doing both simultaneously gets your child further, faster.

Relational therapies can help the brain do some self-assembly and connectivity that might have been lacking in nearly half of children with ASD. At least that is what is shown by Lovass and Sallows, who conclude that nearly 50% of autistic children make significant improvements in behavioral and cognitive skills through behavioral interventions. (See Sallows, *Am.J.Mental Retard* 110 no(6) 2005 p 417-438). I think the 50% who don't recover significantly with behavioral intervention alone may need considerable biomedical intervention before improvement is possible. Of course there are some who just seem beyond reach – at least with what we know today. Still, my advice is to try nutritional intervention together with relational therapy.

STRATEGIES AND PRIORITIES FOR USE OF NUTRITIONAL SUPPLEMENTS FOR ASD

Six Rules for Trials/Use of Nutritional Supplements

I don't know, you don't know, and your assisting health professional doesn't really know which, if any, nutritional supplements will be of benefit and when. But your child or adult with ASD will have responses that will indicate whether you are on the right track or not. I strongly suggest that you keep a diary of what happens with each new trial or change in regimen. This will become a gold mine as time goes on.

1. Use the purest, highest-grade nutritional supplements available. You want complete labeling of all ingredients, active and inactive ("full disclosure"). You need USP quality, pharmaceutical grade, whenever available; Good Manufacturing Practice (GMP) standards followed; FDA compliance on testing for quality and validity of label claims - are all important. Additional analysis proving absence of trace contaminants is very desirable. You want a manufacturer with a track record with the autism community. Remember, one big problem for many with ASD is getting rid of undesirable stuff. You don't want to be putting junk in via supplements.

2. Coordinate supplement trials with the other interventions such as diet trials and medical procedures that your doctor may have underway. Synchronize! If the doctor is trying a medication, hold the nutritional intervention constant and don't make changes until the doctor okays them.

3. Always start with a low amount. You may not see any change, and that's a signal that you could increase the amount and wait for an effect.

4. Discontinue the supplement if there are adverse effects, except in a few cases, such as digestive enzymes or perhaps probiotics, where "worse" may precede "better". But often, worse means worse permanently, so stop the supplement if the worse is much worse or continues unabated. Also, you should discontinue a supplement that worsens a laboratory test result that is related to it. Not all beneficial supplements produce improved behavioral or autistic traits, so I recommend staying with most of those that are included in the Intervention Schedule,

even though their benefits aren't obvious. Supplemental calcium, for example, is required during a dairy-free diet, but you're unlikely to see a behavioral benefit from it.

5. Introduce new supplements one at a time with few exceptions. B_6 and magnesium together is such an exception. Combination products (multivitamins, multiminerals) are a blend of many nutrients, and they can be tried that way. "Super Nu-Thera" (Kirkman) and "Multi-Element Buffered C" (Klaire) are examples of combination products with good track records. If there's a problem, however, there is no way to figure out which ingredient is not tolerated without one-at-a-time ingredient testing. Having to do this is unusual, but it happens.

6. Keep records religiously. What wasn't successful can be as important as what was. Write down the specific symptoms of worsening if it occurs, because you might want a future retrial of that supplement. Don't forget to include amounts and brands in the record.

A Dozen Don't-Dos

There are a lot of ways to do things wrong in this world, and nutritional intervention for ASD is no exception. Many of the published "clinical trials" of nutritional intervention that I've reviewed have failure designed in. Let's not do that here.

1. Don't start two or more different intervention trials at the same time. With diets and supplements, the very minimum time of separation between trial starts is four days. We know this from use of the standard four-day food rotation diet. For some, a seven-day rotation is needed so that food effects don't gang up on limited immune and metabolic tolerances. You may not know whether a food or nutrient supplement is beneficial for the individual until four days have gone by. But you may know a lot sooner if it isn't.

2. Don't begin with detoxification interventions. Most with ASD begin to self-detoxify as soon as toxicant sources are eliminated, non-tolerated foods are removed from the diet, and digestive aids (enzymes) are used. Abruptly adding additional toxicants to the circulation via deliberate detox-specific therapies can cause an overload of circulating toxic junk.

3. Hold off on sophisticated metabolic manipulations until later. Doing them early on is only advisable if you have active medical supervision. Also, I've seen many interventions tried too soon and discarded. Sometimes they might have been very helpful if used later, after preliminary improvements have occurred. Supplementing creatine is an example.

4. Don't use vitamin B_{12} in any form as a separate supplement until you already have L-carnitine in use (acetyl-L-carnitine). Otherwise, you could be wasting a possibly very good supplement because you haven't got its support staff in place.

5. Don't use amino acid supplements (except taurine) until intestinal health has been addressed and dysbiosis has been remedied. What bad bugs in the gut can do with amino acids might, in part, be causative for autism.

6. As stated elsewhere, don't supplement vitamin B_6 without also supplementing magnesium.

7. Don't use supplements that metabolize homocysteine to methionine without having taurine in use. Two such supplements are TMG and DMG. A possible outcome of TMG/DMG use without taurine supplementation is depletion of taurine in the CNS and (worsened) seizures.

8. Don't rely on laboratory tests of urine analytes for guidance on supplementation when analytes are ratioed to creatinine and creatinine itself is subnormal. Slightly low creatinine is commonly seen in ASD. Dividing a low analyte level by a low creatinine level gives a false normal result. If creatinine is very low, renal clearance may be a problem. This is rare in ASD, but I've seen it a few times. No nutritional supplements should be used without close medical supervision if kidney clearance isn't normal.

9. If your ASD individual has excessive urine levels of oxalate, be sure that calcium and lipase (a digestive enzyme) are supplemented, as well as taurine, vitamin B_6, and magnesium. Many mineral supplements use glycine-complexed elements. For some who are genetically predisposed, too much glycine leads to internal formation of oxalate.

10. At supper or in the evening, don't give supplements that contain phenylalanine, tyrosine, or histidine, and don't feed high-protein meals late in the day. Doing this reduces tryptophan transport into the brain with consequent limitation on serotonin and melatonin. Insomnia is likely then, as is poor rejuvenation of cell function, lessened immune defense, decreased detoxication and sustained inflammation.

11. Don't use cysteine, cystine, or alpha-lipoic acid as nutritional supplements except under medical supervision and with periodic checks of intestinal yeast content.

12. Don't use N-acetylcysteine unless it is certified to be the reduced, active form, and then do periodic checks of intestinal yeast content. Unfortunately, most over-the-counter NAC contains oxidized material. For both 11 and 12, be especially careful if the individual is hypothyroid.

Supplement Intervention Schedule

A good way to understand how to go from being lost in the woods to arriving home is to have a map with identified landmarks. A better way might be with a directional GPS with verbal prompts, but we're a long way from having that for ASD. So, I've provided the best map (schedule) I know for you. Later on in this book, you'll find a descriptive text for each nutrient/supplement that's listed in the schedule. In this section, after the schedule, there's a descriptive text for each "tier" of intervention. Doing intervention trials in this order minimizes problems – in my experience. Of course, a health professional may guide you toward a different schedule if there's a good reason to do so. With all the individuality in ASD, variance from what I've set out isn't necessarily wrong and may be a shortcut. In any case, I hope there's significant improvement as you move along. Some parents have gone through this with good outcomes in as little as six months. Sometimes with setbacks and relapses, two years is required to give it a fair trial. Best wishes to all.

Preliminaries and Prerequisites

      Diagnosis of ASD

      Find a qualified doctor or physician assistant

      Find a qualified nutrition counselor

      Record patient and family histories

      Environmental cleanup

      Diet cleanup

      Arrange for relational therapy

Initial tests

- Physical exam
- Blood chemistry, CBC
- Thyroid markers
- Urinalysis
- Stool analysis including digestive and inflammation markers, microbiology, mycology and parasitology
- Blood ammonia?
- Other doctor-ordered tests
- Metric tests of autism severity

If urinalysis shows stones, high urate or high oxalate, follow doctor/s and/or nutrition counselor's recommendations. High urate suggests need for low purine diet; high oxalate is an indication for a low oxalate diet. If ammonia is high, follow doctor recommendations. Appropriate nutritional measures for elevated ammonia include lowered dietary protein, use of alpha-ketoglutaric acid (buffered supplement), and anti-intestinal-dysbiosis measures

TIER 1, Basic for ASD, CF Trial
Digestive aids (enzymes)
Alpha-ketoglutarate if ammonia is elevated
Activated charcoal (use as needed)
Calcium, magnesium, multiminerals?
Taurine
L-carnitine
Multivitamins: B complex, folate, A,C,D,E
Melatonin
Omega-3 Fatty acids

TIER 2, Intestinal Cleanup, GF Trial
Continue Tier 1 supplements, plus
Herbal antibiotics: oregano, thyme
Activated charcoal
Probiotics & S. boulardii
Turmeric, silymarin
More antioxidant nutrients?
Zinc
Carnosine, esp. with seizure cases

TIER 3, Healing Period, Carbohydrate check, Gut check
More Omega-3 fatty acids
Continue Tier 1 supplements; perhaps more L-carnitine
Continue but reduce Tier 2 supplements to
maintenance levels for intestinal health
If oxalate was high initially, retest now. If still high,
check fat content of stool with new stool analysis;
Recheck intestinal flora and digestive markers

TIER 4, Detox and Antioxidant Brigade
Continue supplements as in Tier 3, plus
Extra vitamin C
Glutathione, NAC
Extra taurine
Magnesium malate
CoQ10
Watch out for reoccurrence of dysbiosis

TIER 5, Special Metabolic Measures
Continue supplements as in Tier 3
Continue Tier 4 detox and antioxidant
Supplements at reduced or maintenance levels, plus:
Creatine
Amino Acids
DMG or TMG, folinic acid
Methylcobalamin
Carnosine (may have been tried in Tier 2)
Bacopa

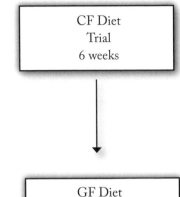

CF Diet
Trial
6 weeks

GF Diet
Trial
12-16 weeks

Try or continue
Low Oxalate
Diet?

Choose and stay on
most beneficial diet
Detoxification therapies
– chelation,
saunas, sulfate baths
clean environment
is essential.

Continue Diet

~ Tier Explanations ~

Intervention Schedule – Preliminaries

You want a doctor who has some experience in dealing with gastrointestinal issues, toxicology and detoxification, immune dysfunction, allergy and inflammation, and who understands the value of nutritional therapy. Also, your doctor should be one who connects well with other important disciplines such as dietary adjustment and relational therapy. Ask other parents for suggestions; ask your nutrition counselor if you've got one; call ARI or TACA or local support organizations. If you use the Internet, try to get five or ten minutes of actual "interview" time on the phone before traveling a long distance for the first appointment.

A complete patient (and family) history provided to your doctor will save time, help to prevent wasted efforts and provide clues as to what interventions have the best outcome possibilities.

You may need immediate dietary counseling that goes beyond what your doctor is able to advise on. Nutrition textbooks usually cover special diets (low purine, low oxalate, low protein). If you think you need this, get help from a registered or licensed nutrition counselor who knows the details.

Progress Assessment Metrics

I advise use of initial, periodic and outcome assessment measures as an unbiased way of gauging progress. Sometimes called "metrics", there are many tests to choose from and doing more than one is fine. Just be consistent and do the same ones as you go along. Of course, you're measuring the whole program's effects – nutritional intervention including diet, your doctor's treatments, relational therapy and special education sessions. Later on, you'll be glad you did this.

ATEC, Autism Treatment Evaluation Checklist

One-page questionnaire for 5-12 year olds that records status of: speech and communication, social interaction, sensory awareness, cognitive ability, behavior and physical health. You can use the ARI website (www.autism.com) for scoring.

ADOS, Autism Diagnostic Observation Schedule

This one is administered by a trained professional, and it applies to children and adults. A favorite assessment tool, the ADOS scores sociability, communication skills, and behavior.

CARS, Childhood Autism Rating Scale

Usually done by your doctor or health professional, it applies to children above 24 months of age. The clinician rates the child's abilities in 15 areas based on criteria set by the test.

GARS, Gilliam Autism Rating Scale (GARS II, 2006)

This is a series of 42 parent-answered questions that applies for ages 3 to 22 years. Sociability, communication and stereotypical behaviors are graded against a sample group of autistic children. The score indicates the level of the tested individual relative for "average" for autism.

CARD used by the Center for Autism Related Disorders (Granpeesheh D, et al., A.S.Q. version 2007) to assess the level of autism symptoms and traits and measure status/improvement before and during applied behavioral analysis (ABA). ABA is an excellent form of relational therapy.

There are at least half a dozen other assessment measurements that could be used, including GADS for those with Asperger's Disorder. You may find more information on this from local support groups.

Intervention Schedule – Tier 1

This is a trial of basic supplements for ASD together with a casein-free (CF) diet trial. In reality, it is also phase 1 of intestinal cleanup. More overt and aggressive cleanup occurs in Tier 2, but this is something that's best done in stages, not all at once.

Begin with digestive enzymes and don't be surprised by temporarily worsened behaviors, new, aberrant behaviors, irritability, and what might be a headache (if only they could talk!). Bowel movements may change in timing and stool appearance. Activated charcoal to the rescue, if necessary. Don't worry about the resulting charcoal-blackened stools. What is happening is that bowel flora is changing because there is less undigested food for them to feed on. There may be die-off of some species, which will cause temporarily higher levels of the chemicals they produce. Be sure dipeptidylpeptidase IV (DPP4) activity is included in the digestive enzyme supplement.

If elevated blood ammonia is diagnosed, an appropriate nutritional aid is supplementation of (buffered) alpha-ketoglutarate. Follow your doctor's instructions about what else to do. Besides helping with excess ammonia, A-Kg aids mitochondrial energy and antioxidant processes, so it can be supplemented to those purposes continually or during any tier of intervention.

After a week or ten days, begin the casein-free diet. This needs to be as perfect as possible – 100% exclusion of casein. Consult with a nutritionist, read books, get local help if available. Be sure to read food packaging labels. "Caseinates" are casein forms. Unfortunately, sometimes casein is added to processed foods and it's not necessarily on the label. At least five out of ten (50%) of autistic children improve gradually in behavior (some quickly) with casein avoidance. But many first go through a withdrawal period. Casomorphins (undigested casein-source peptides) are addictive. Their removal causes an opiate-like withdrawal, often with temporary worsening of autistic behaviors.

A dairy-free diet almost always goes too low in calcium for children. So the next thing is supplementation of calcium, and I advise co-supplementation of magnesium, in a ratio of 2 or 3 parts calcium to 1 part magnesium. If you're giving 400 mg of calcium, then also give 130 to 200 mg of magnesium. This ratio is a little higher in magnesium than standard nutrition calls for, but you may need it as soon as you put in B_6 with the other vitamins. Magnesium malate is a supplement form that you may wish to try now. It's called for later on in the schedule (Tier 4).

Next comes taurine, then carnitine, probably as acetyl-L-carnitine. Next, try a multivitamin. Some of these products come with magnesium included, some don't. If yours does, then maybe back off on the other magnesium supplement so that you don't exceed one part magnesium to two parts calcium. Extra magnesium is rapidly excreted in the urine, but loose stools and too-frequent bowel movements can result from extra amounts. If your child is on lithium therapy, as some with autism are, then a higher ratio of calcium-to-magnesium such as 4 to 1, may be required to keep blood lithium in the therapeutic range. However, don't go above 5 to 1 Ca to Mg.

Melatonin comes next. If sleep is an issue, melatonin helps, and it's also a natural anti-inflammation agent. You should review the Circadian Rhythm text in the Appendix as well as the chapter on melatonin. Not only does it promote sleep and anti-inflammatory actions, it helps cells to organize their nightly cleanup efforts. The importance of this cannot be overstated. Neither biochemistry nor behavior can be made right without sleep.

The last nutritional supplement in this tier is the essential, long-chain fatty acids, especially the omega-3 type. With taurine and lipase (in the digestive enzymes) in place as supplements, both the fatty acids and the lipid-soluble vitamins (A,D,E) should be well absorbed.

If you've tried these nutritional supplements and introduced them one at a time, then you're probably into the 4th or 5th week of the CF diet trial. Stay where you are on supplements for another week so that the diet has been given six weeks to work.

Next, you have to decide whether to abandon this diet and go on to a trial of the gluten-free diet, or whether to stay with it while going gluten-free, too. For most, the choice will be clear. If you're uncertain and want to challenge with a glass of milk followed in four hours with a dish of (natural) vanilla ice cream, be sure your spouse, brother/sister, adult helper is on hand. If nothing happens, fine, casein is something you don't have to worry about. If you do get a reaction, the supplements will help to alleviate it, especially the digestive enzymes, melatonin and taurine. However, a reaction to casein-containing food means that you stick to the CF diet and wait ten more days before starting Tier 2.

Intervention Schedule, Tier 2

Here's where we kill off bad flora that's still in the gut, populate it with good flora, and determine if gluten foods are causing problems. You should continue the supplements that helped or for which there was no adverse response per the Tier 1 experiences. You may or may not be continuing with the casein-free diet as well. Yes, there are very likely to be bacterial spores, morphed forms of yeast, and resistant and resourceful dysbiotic flora still present despite the Tier 1 efforts. These may be the same culprits that survive and thrive after standard antibiotic treatments for infections. Once these culprits have dug in, you're not very likely to get rid of them with dietary restrictions alone.

I suggest going on the gluten free diet for a week before calling in the "hired guns" of nutrition to eliminate dysbiotic flora. When you do put them to work, it's for 30 days along with friendly (probiotic) flora, some of which will sustain collateral damage from the hired guns. Your doctor is in charge of which, if any, anti-yeast and/or antibacterial medicinal agents are used. The nutritional guns are two antibacterial herbals and one yeast that kills other yeasts. The herbals are thyme and oregano (in capsule form), the killer yeast is Saccharomyces boulardii. The herbals are described in the section on Herbals. You'll want some protective shields when these are used: activated charcoal, turmeric (capsule form) and silymarin. Use of these is also explained later.

Probiotic use is essential in concert with with and continuing after the brigade of dysbiotic-flora killers. You can wait a week or two before introducing probiotic supplements, but not longer than that. It's true, some of these good guys will get killed off along with the harmful flora; that's unavoidable. But you've got to get the good guys implanted and colonized before you stop using the herbals, S. boulardii and medicinal antibiotics (if any). According to parents I've talked with, giving the killers in the AM and the probiotics (between meals with water) in the PM has worked well. The probiotics to use are described in the probiotic chapter and include types of lactobacillus and Bifidobacter bifidum.

Can you test out of this part of Tier 2? I remember in graduate school passing a two-day battery of qualifying exams that allowed me to skip a master's degree and go directly into Ph.D. studies in chemical engineering. I soon found the Ph.D. coursework damn hard and wondered why I decided to do that. Invariably, tests do not test everything you're supposed to know about a subject. Well, your ASD person may test out of intestinal cleanup if he/she can show by analytical tests that there's no evidence of excess yeast and that aerobic gut bacteria are normal according to stool analyses, plus showing normalcy for urine markers for yeast and for anerobic bacteria like clostridia. These urine markers include IAG, DHPPA, and others as offered by Great Plains, Genova, and MetaMetrix Laboratories. But in my opinion, even if all of these tests are negative for intestinal dysbiosis, I'd still do the hired-gun and shield routine for two weeks. Why? Well, what if clostridia were present, went to spore form and hid out while the testing was done? In that event, you'd never know it was there during the testing.

Zinc may have been included in a Tier 1 multimineral supplement. If so, fine. Try it after you're as sure as you can be that digestive aids are working, foods aren't causing intestinal inflammation and neither are dysbiotic flora. Not all with ASD have subnormal zinc levels in blood or cells, but some do. Attempting to normalize zinc levels with oral supplements is just frustrating if you don't have the gastrointestinal tract in good shape. Also, essential fatty acid supplements beforehand (in Tier 1) help with normalizing blood cell zinc levels. Much of the zinc measured by lab tests on unwashed ("packed") blood cell specimens is surface zinc bound to membrane fatty acids. Mildly low blood cell zinc usually means there's a membrane fatty acid/zinc problem. Significantly low cell zinc means it's low inside too.

Carnosine metabolism requires zinc, and carnosine is the last nutritional supplement to be tried in Tier 2. Please read the carnosine section first. This supplement is one you should stay with only if it helps. If you don't see a beneficial effect after a week or ten days, I recommend discontinuing it. That's because the beta-alanine, which is part of carnosine, acts to increase urinary loss of taurine, and that may have undesirable consequences. If carnosine helps, then use it and increase the daily taurine supplement by 30 to 50%.

After 12 to 16 weeks on Tier 2, it's time to decide if the gluten-free diet helped. Typically, the "help" is less obvious than is the effect of casein avoidance. That's one reason why the gluten avoidance trial is at least twice as long as the casein one. Again, two challenge meals about four hours apart usually tell the tale if you are otherwise undecided. Have help handy. If there's no reason to continue the GF diet, that's good news – one less complication. But if you do get a reaction from the challenge meals, then it's at least two weeks back on the GF diet before you can do a valid trial of anything else.

Intervention Schedule, Tier 3

During Tier 3 we're going to give the intestinal tract a healing period unless there's evidence of intestinal distress, food reactivity or digestion problems. If the CF and/or GF diets have been beneficial and progress is being made, then continue with that as long as there is progress. If you're uncertain about intestinal status, do another stool analysis. A urine organic acid analysis that includes dysbiosis markers can be ordered to assess status of some of the intestinal anerobic organisms.

If the CF and/or GF diets did not bring about satisfactory improvements and there still are symptoms of intestinal distress, perhaps the specific carbohydrate diet is the answer. The SCD is more limited, but it is very useful for some. Because of its limitations, it can't very well be combined with other diets (e.g. low oxalate). Trying to do so would probably not leave enough food or food diversity for a healthy diet. Also, with perhaps three in ten, diet does not seem to be the problem. However, the only feasible way to know that is to try the diets.

Just as with the CF and GF diets, digestive aid use is a big assist with the SCD. But that's only if the digestive supplement contains enzymes that digest carbohydrates and complex sugars. Maltase, isomaltase and sucrase are some of the enzymes which go after the complex sugars that the SCD is designed to minimize. Neither the enzyme supplements nor the diet is perfect, and doing both is the best course.

If your ASD individual had elevated oxalate in urine, and whether or not you've been using a low oxalate diet, now it's time to recheck that with a lab test. Improved digestion, use of probiotic supplements, use of taurine and calcium supplements, together with the other measures that you have kept as beneficial, may have solved the oxalate problem. If not, then again consult with your nutrition counselor about use of a low oxalate diet.

Increasing the daily supplement of omega-3 fatty acids (docosahexaenoic, eicosapentaenoic, alpha-linolenic) can be beneficial at this time.

Intervention Schedule, Tier 4

Now is the time to purge remaining toxicants from body tissues and get the body's own detoxication processes revved up. To do this, you'll also need to get more antioxidant protection in place. Hopefully, by now you either have settled on the best dietary intervention, based on behavioral and analytical evidence, or you've concluded that a special diet isn't needed. However, I wouldn't be too quick to discontinue digestive aid use. The enzymes may actually be helping with food tolerance and now isn't a good time to discontinue them. That's something you might try at the very end of this whole intervention schedule (after Tier 5 activities).

Continue all the supplements that provided behavioral and cognitive benefit, or that are likely to be of nutritional benefit. One at a time, add into the daily regimen:
- More vitamin C, not to exceed 2.0 grams/day of ascorbate (a multi-element buffered form of vitamin C is best) for older children and teens, and not more than one gram/day for younger children (2-4 years of age).
- Reduced glutathione (GSH). Mostly, oral GSH increases intestinal antioxidant activity. However, some of it is absorbed intact. Up to 500 mg/day usually works well, 250 mg/d for young children.
- N-acetylcysteine, up to 250 mg/d, but watch out for development of intestinal yeast overgrowth. Continue periodic, low-dose S. boulardii. Herbals like olive leaf extract and oregano, and caprylic acid (is a type of fatty acid) can be used

to suppress intestinal yeast overgrowth that might be encouraged by NAC or GSH. Ensure that the NAC is not oxidized material.

- Taurine at 500 to 1000 mg/d, for older children, and 250 to 500 for younger children, as total daily supplemental amount, is usually well tolerated and helpful during Tier 4 .
- Magnesium malate works directly at reducing mitochondrial oxidant stress. Most formulations provide two magnesium atoms to one of malate, and about 1000 mg of the product per day is helpful (200 mg of magnesium; the remainder is the malate). Use about half this for young children and reduce other magnesium supplements so as not to exceed 1 part Mg to 2 parts Ca.
- CoQ10 at up to 100 mg/day also helps mitochondrial function.

While you are doing this, you should be coordinating closely with your doctor if he/she is also doing detoxification therapies, like chelation or sauna. Something you can try at home is magnesium sulfate baths. Put ten or twelve cups of Epsom salts in warm bath water and bathe the child (or adult), and periodically add warm water so the bath lasts about 15 minutes. Eventually, longer baths (up to 30 mins) can be beneficial. Sweating during the baths is better still. I'm told that the reason for this gradual process is that, ideally, lots of toxicants come out early on, so it's better in the beginning to get out of the water sooner. You'll have to buy the large cartons of Epsom salts (OTC, drugstore or grocery store) to do this. Most package directions will say two cups per gallon of water. I think one cup per gallon works fine. Just a few cups of mag sulfate per bath won't do much and you are wasting the salt by using too little. A standard bathtub, with 4-5 inches of water in it and the child, contains about 12 gallons of water.

I cannot overstress the importance of a clean, toxicant-free environment during Tier 4 and from then on. Some children with ASD self-detox after Tier 3 or during Tier 4 without purposeful detoxification procedures.

Intervention Schedule, Tier 5

At this point, basic nutrition has been bolstered, the intestinal tract should be in better shape with proper flora and digestion, sequestered toxicants have been mostly removed from body tissues, and cells are better able to do energy conversions and assemble molecules that are needed for physical and mental processes. If necessary, a diet that excludes troublemaking foods is in place, and you have done your best to provide a clean environment. Additionally, you are doing relational therapy and special education activities that improve neuronal network abilities for perception, memory and response. You're continuing, to give maintenance levels of supplements that defend the body against toxic and infectious stressors, and most importantly, you're likely to have reduced inflammation very significantly. Now, it's time to try some special supplements – those that might further improve cellular energy output, transport processes, methylation and neuronal communication.

The six supplement items listed in the Tier 5 section of the schedule might be tried in almost any order. I prefer to start with creatine because it's our energy-delivery agent. No matter what else we improve, energy delivery to neurons has to be adequate or expressive speech will remain inhibited. Please read or review the chapter on creatine before beginning, and be sure you've got a quality supplement. This is because, if it helps, it usually does so in gram quantities per day. At these levels, even small impurities will add up. Start with 100 mg/kg (about 50 mg/lb), body weight and be prepared to go to 500 mg/kg (250 mg/lb) or higher. Doctors have used as much as 1000 mg or 1.0 gram per kg in children and 2000 mg/kg in adults without notable side effects. The chances of creatine helping are small, 5 to 10% at most. But the help, if it comes, is with vastly increased responses to environmental happenings, expressive speech, perhaps some hyperactivity or at least lots of energy to which you will have to adjust. The responses, for a few, have been likened to a spring-powered toy that's suddenly wound up, become unrestrained, and is making a commotion. If this is going to happen, it does so in about a week or less. If you don't see anything after two weeks, then it's time to give it up and start to work on methylation.

Supplements that directly help with methylation include DMG, TMG, folinic acid, and methylcobalamin. What we're trying to do here is improve the synchrony of neuronal networks by improving methylation of membrane lipids adjacent to receptors in neurons. Neurons and neuronal networks don't work in synchrony if they are energy-starved (a creatine deficiency problem); and they also don't work in synchrony if they don't have adequate flexibility and signal-transmitting ability (methylation-dependent properties). Methylation is provided by S-adenosylmethionine, SAM. Many of the methylation problems in autism stem from impaired homocysteine-to-methionine metabolism. See the Glossary for more information on this. Simply put, we tried the energy route (creatine) to improvement first. If that didn't help, next we'll try the material-supply route (methyls).

Methylated vitamin B_{12} (methylcobalamin) is best administered by injection, a medical procedure that is beyond the scope of this book. Consult your doctor. I'm told that use of the nasal spray cobalamin also is a medical procedure that works, but is somewhat less effective than injectable methylcobalamin for our purposes. That's not to say it wouldn't work well for your child, because it might, and it's a procedure that avoids needle-sticking.

You may have already included some oral methylcobalamin in the regimen back in Tier 1 with use of a multivitamin supplement. You can now try an extra amount as a stand-alone supplement at "mega-dose" level to see if that helps. If you're also giving vitamin C or ascorbate, it's best to give the cobalamin at a different mealtime. Powders and capsules containing methylcobalamin are available, and a daily amount (serving) of 1000 to 5000 mcg (micrograms) for about three or four weeks should be long enough to tell if it's helping. You're looking for a decrease in the autistic traits of isolation, poor interactions, lack of speech, and for an improvement in processing sensory inputs.

DMG is dimethylglycine and TMG is its metabolic precursor, trimethylglycine. TMG comes from dietary lecithin and body-made choline. Choline now is classed as nutritionally essential, and both DMG and TMG are active, daughter forms of choline. They are methyl sources when they come into the body as food. Please read or review the chapter on DMG and TMG before using either.

Start with DMG because it provokes the lesser amount of adverse responses (8%, n=6363 per ARI Publ. 34, 2009). TMG provokes adverse responses in 16%, n=1132, per the same parent survey.

It's okay to give DMG with methylcobalamin and/or with folinic acid, and the same is true for TMG. However, parents have not reported on use of DMG and TMG together, although I don't see a problem with that either. TMG methylates homocysteine directly to make methionine; the TMG becomes DMG in doing so. DMG does not directly methylate homocysteine. Instead, the DMG molecule comes apart producing "one-carbon" chemical pieces which become methyls that make methyltetrahydrofolate. MethylTHF gives the methyl to cobalamin and that gives the methyl to homocysteine, again making methionine. The amounts of DMG and TMG to try are listed in the descriptive chapter. Just be sure you're still providing a taurine supplement when you do the DMG and TMG trials. As with methylcobalamin, you're looking for further improvement in core autistic traits: lack of interaction, lack of speech; and for improvement in processing news from the outside.

Sometimes there's notable improvement with DMG or TMG, but there's also increased hyperactivity. That's often toned down with added folic acid. I have a slight preference for use of folinic acid which, for our purposes, gives somewhat better options and outcomes biochemically. You might try folic acid with DMG or TMG; many parents swear by it. Others prefer DMG or TMG with folinic acid. Both folic and folinic acid forms of folate supplements are described in the vitamin chapter. I do not advise use of stand-alone folic acid supplements. My experience with use of just folic acid is that, by itself, it too often results in worsened autistic traits. Folinic acid seems to avoid this, usually, but not always.

Up to this point we have focused on making the body operational for self-synthesis of what it needs. Now, let's see if supplementing the supply of raw materials will be of benefit. It's time to try amino acid supplements. The body uses amino acids to make creatine, carnitine, glutathione, melatonin, thyroid hormones, taurine, digestive enzymes, etc. Please read or review the amino acid chapter before proceeding.

As explained in that chapter, there are two ways to go about this. The least expensive way is to try a prepared blend of essential and protein amino acids, probably one that includes some taurine as well, and follow label instructions or those of your doctor or nutrition counselor. The second way is to try to match individual needs by doing a quantitative blood or 24-hour urine analysis with a clinical laboratory that also provides a calculated supplement formula. Have the doctor send that formula to a compounding pharmacy that will make up an individualized blend of amino acids as called for by the formula. Obviously, this second way is considerably more expensive. I suggest that you try amino acid supplements for a month unless you run into reactivities, behavioral regression or other symptoms of intolerance. Approximately half of autistic children show some benefit from amino acid supplements at this stage – per anecdotal reports to me. If you do run into problems, stop the supplement, and, if possible, have the doctor send blood plasma or a 24-hour urine specimen to a clinical lab for amino acid analysis. You may then uncover a hidden-until-now problem with metabolism. While this is quite uncommon, I've consulted on a few dozen such cases over the years. Problems with amino acid supplements are much more likely to be due to intestinal dysbiosis which has crept in unnoticed and with symptoms that become overt when amino acids are present. A stool analysis or a urine organic acid analysis with dysbiosis markers should tell the tale. You also have to be sure that L-carnitine and vitamin B_{12} are doing their work in cell mitochondria, because amino acid metabolism naturally leads to products that have to be processed inside cell mitochondria.

Amino acid supplements can bring about wonderful improvements, but they require fully operational cell chemistry. This is why we don't try amino acids until this time in the intervention schedule. If you should experience some regression with amino acid supplements, discontinuing them relieves such problems after a few days. Also, alpha-ketoglutaric acid (buffered), acetyl-L-carnitine, and B-vitamins, given with lots of pure water, usually hasten recovery from amino acid-caused symptoms. The chances are good that you won't have such symptoms. Also, there's about a fifty-fifty chance that you won't see noticeable improvement with amino acid supplements. If so, dietary protein intake and digestion are doing an adequate job, and that's even better!

There's one last item I can suggest, the herb, bacopa (Bacopa monniere), which you may find at a local health food store. This herb was brought to my attention by Robert Elghammer, MD, of Danville IL. We know each other through the Academy of Environmental Medicine (formerly Clinical Ecology). His father, Robert Elghammer MD (senior, now deceased) by coincidence was my pediatrician. Way ahead of his time, he got me off foods I didn't tolerate when I was four years old. Dr. Robert (junior) has used bacopa for years in his pediatric practice and noticed its particular benefit for ASD children and told me about it.

For some, bacopa improves memory, learning speed and mental endurance. It's available in gelatin capsules usually containing 100 mg of bacopa plant substances including "bacosides". 100 to 200 mg/d is the amount to try; hopefully you'll see good things in about two weeks. It has been used for at least 3000 years beginning in India; there are recent scientific studies (1997-present) that indicate cognitive improvements and other benefits with its use. More information is available online.

TECHNICAL INFORMATION ON
NUTRITIONAL SUPPLEMENTS

Legal Status

The US Food and Drug Administration (FDA) is the government agency that oversees and regulates manufacture and sales of nutritional supplements. An important governing law is "DSHEA", the Dietary Supplement Health and Education Act (1994); it covers safety, product labeling and claims, manufacturing practices and FDA authority. All nutritional supplements are, by law, classed as food – not medicine. Even capsules of activated charcoal, which might help to negate the effects of intestinal toxicants, are sold as food – so there's quite a bit of latitude allowed for what a supplement can be. Not so for advertising or claims.

Allowable Claims

Medical or curative claims for nutritional supplements are only rarely allowed. That's when the nutrient has overwhelming clinical evidence that's widely accepted by medical professionals that a curative property exists. Vitamin C preventing and helping to cure scurvy is an example. A probiotic alleviating colitis would not be an allowable claim.

What's generally allowed are valid "form and function" claims by manufacturers and vendors. Form refers to the physical and chemical description of the nutrients in the product. Function is what textbooks and/or authoritative published research document the nutrient to do physiologically in the body. A manufacturer can, for example, say that vitamin C enhances formation of L-carnitine, because that is a biochemical action which it does (New *Eng J Med* 314, no 14, p 893). But the manufacturer cannot say that vitamin C helps to alleviate some types of autism – even though the logic seems correct.

That brings up the issue of who can say what. I can say what I believe or know to be true – it's my First Amendment right. I'm not a manufacturer and I'm not compensated by one and I won't be in the future. While the manufacturer/marketer of nutritional supplements is generally not allowed to make medical claims for nutrient products, independent researchers can. Such findings might be published if the researchers are experienced or credentialed professionals and if the research follows correct scientific methods. Even so, a manufacturer/marketer may often be unable to use such published findings as advertising claims. That's because a whole lot of time, money, and legal muscle would be required. An unfortunate consequence is that manufacturers usually do not do controlled clinical studies to demonstrate curative or preventative efficacy of nutritional supplements. They'd be spending hugely for something they can't legally use and likely couldn't patent or enforce ownership rights to.

That leaves you three resources to go to, to learn about nutritional supplements beyond form and function –

1. Consult your doctor or qualified health professional
2. Take college courses in biochemistry, physiology and medicine and then read the published scientific/medical articles on supplements of interest
3. Survey other parents for their experience with use of nutritional supplements – in our case, for ASD.

Resourse (1) is best, (2) costs lots of money and takes forever, and (3) is good but may be diluted with misinformation and experiences that don't apply to the individual's needs. There is a quick way to do option (3) by looking at ARI Publication 34 (latest editions) and playing the odds: www.autism.com. If a supplement or strategy seems to work for a substantial number of people, it's worth trying to see if it will work for your family member. There is a copy of 2009 Publ. 34 in the Appendix.

Safety and Purity of Nutritional Supplements

If you want the facts on deaths and reported illness caused by nutritional supplement use versus those caused by "ethical" drugs, you can visit several websites or information services –

- US Food and Drug Administration, Center for Food Safety and Applied Nutrition
- PubMed Central – Injury Prevention: www.ncbi.nlm.nih.gov/pmc/articles
- Natural News.com, see www.naturalnews.com/027993
- Orthomolecular.org, see www.orthomolecular.org/resources/omni/vo4n13.shtml

For the year 2009 (the latest year that I have complete data for), there were zero deaths attributed to nutritional supplement use: US National Poison Data System as quoted by *Natural News*, Jan 21, 2010. For 2008, there were five (5) deaths, 85 hospitalizations and about 600 "adverse events" per www.orthomolecular.org. However, reading the fine print reveals that almost all of these events, including deaths and hospitalizations, were attributed to weight-loss products or to stuff taken by bodybuilders. What stuff? Gamma-hydroxybutyrate (GHB), 1,4-butanediol (BD), gamma-butyrolactone (GBL); that kind of stuff. That's NOT what we're talking about for nutritional intervention in ASD.

Now, how are the pharmaceuticals doing? Honestly, that's a safety disaster area. *Natural News* states that on the order of 100,000 deaths occur each year with use of FDA-approved medicines – per the *Journal of the American Medical Association* (JAMA). The FDA acknowledges 482,154 adverse-event reports for 2007 – www.orthomolecular.org. For ICD code data, we have to go back in time to 2002-03 when about 25,000 deaths had prescription drugs listed as the primary cause per Pub Med – www.ncbi.nlm.nih.gov/pubmed/17536879. And from this same reference, guess what medication-associated death had the highest percentage increase between 1999 and 2003. Answer – antibiotic-related

Clostridium difficile enterocolitis. This is the colitis that can be caused by excessive use of fluoroquinolone-type antibiotics, vancomycin and the cephalosporins, especially when appropriate probiotic supplements are not also used.

Does this mean that the nutritional supplements that I'm describing for ASD should get a "clean bill of health"? No way – unfortunately. During the last decade, foreign sources of nutrient materials became increasingly available at relatively cheap cost. It used to be just the herbals from China, India and the Far East that we worried about. But during the last decade, more foreign sourcing of raw materials has occurred. I'm informed that now the majority of raw materials for nutritional supplement manufacture comes from foreign sources, a lot of it from places where "quality control" is a recent and unwelcome nuisance. Much of this stuff comes from China – where lead-painted toys and toxic pet food originated. And I'm also told by knowledgeable people that these imported materials are "hit-or-miss" when it comes to both assay and contaminant problems. One batch might be fine; the next one very much not so.

By assay, I mean potency that meets (or exceeds) label claims. Assay variance from label claims will be known before the product is marketed if the manufacturer adheres to new FDA requirements for analytical testing of ingredient content. If the material isn't 95% vitamin X, for example, the batch can be rejected and the supplier directed to provide one that meets specifications. All US supplement manufacturers are or will soon be required to do this so that label claims of content are valid.

Not so easy – screening out batches with trace contaminants that may be harmful to consumers and probably would be harmful to the ASD population. Please realize that meeting label claims for potency does not assure that potentially harmful contaminants are absent. DDT (outlawed in the US for decades) dicofol (its near-twin replacement) and other organochlorine and organophosphate spray residues should be analyzed for. Also, trace and not-so-trace levels of mercury, lead, arsenic, antimony and chromium +6 need to be guarded against. That's because the typical victim of ASD just doesn't detoxify as well as a normal person can. Daily input of trace toxicants leads to an accumulation of stuff that reinforces the maladapted metabolism we find in many with autism. What about bacteria or their spores in herbals? Are we going to be on guard for this as well? We ought to. We should hold supplement manufacturers to the highest possible standards of quality. I urge you, as parents and clinicians, to purchase nutritional supplements on the basis of quality – not cost.

There is only one manufacturer of nutritional supplements that I know of that markets to parents and caregivers for ASD and now is doing detailed testing for trace levels of agricultural chemicals (crop sprays) including organochlorines and organophosphates, toxic elements, and microorganisms– for each and every lot of product. That manufacturer is Kirkman Laboratories of Lake Oswego, Oregon. They promise written certification of analysis upon request. Also, Kirkman Labs plans to indemnify doctors who purchase Kirkman products against contaminant problems of this nature. This is the only commercial in this book. If you represent or know of any manufacturer that matches this capability, send me written documentation of such, and I'll include that manufacturer's name in the next edition of this book (if I am the author). I receive no compensation of any kind from Kirkman or from any other provider of nutritional supplements.

Synthetics

Let's start by dispelling the misconception that natural is always good and synthetic is bad. Synthetic doesn't mean it's different; it means it's synthesized – man made. Usually, in nutrition, natural is better, but that's not necessarily true when it comes to essential nutrients at trace or milligram levels. Why? There are three reasons.

First, obtaining the desired nutrient for supplement manufacturing (vitamin, amino acid, element, other metabolic factor) requires that physical, chemical, thermal and some-times electrical processes be used to concentrate the one part that is desired from the many other parts of natural material. Doing so alters the natural ingredients. If it were just a matter of filtering, there would be no problem. But it's not. Distillation, a sometimes-used thermal process, can harm heat-labile nutrients like vitamins A or C, and may partially oxidize important antioxidants like vitamin E. Chemical extraction, often used in nutrient manufacture, involves adding a chemical, like alcohol, to separate the desired nutrient by dissolving it away from the non-soluble part of the natural substance. Then the alcohol and all of its impurities have to be gotten rid of, as well as whatever else got dissolved.

The second problem that has to be overcome is the presence of residual levels of agri-cultural and animal-treatment chemicals that may be in the raw materials. These chemicals could be pesticides, herbicides, fungicides, growth or ripening modifiers, hormones, antibi-otics, etc. The obvious answer to this is to use only organically-grown crops or livestock as raw material sources. Do all supplement manufacturers do this? If you're determined to use only all-natural nutritional supplements, you might ask for written certification that only legally-organic raw material was used – good luck!

Finally, there are the allergy problems that some of us have and that seem to me to be more prevalent in the ASD population. Corn allergy, if severe, can cause problems with most "natural-source" vitamin C; it's mostly made from corn. "Rose-hip" vitamin C? All the manufacturer needs for a product to be called that is to include 5% (or more) rose hip-source ascorbate in the product. The rest can be corn-source ascorbate. If the ASD individual has a corn allergy, try to find synthetic ascorbate or the 99.9% pure grade. Much of the vitamin C powder that's used for supplement purposes is only 95% pure ascorbic acid or ascorbate salt such as calcium ascorbate. What's the rest? It's mostly cornstarch. Allergen carry-over into nutritional supplement products has been a problem for as long as I can remember, and sometimes natural impurities are more than just allergens – casein and gluten are examples.

One vitamin that seems better tolerated by some with ASD when it's synthetic is vitamin E. Natural vitamin E is an oil also made by chemically processing corn. Natural vitamin E does have the advantage of containing the various tocopherols that make up the vitamin E family of tocopherols. That's fine if there's no corn allergy and if the person can detoxify whatever else carries through the production process.

Synthetic L-form amino acids are far better in terms of purity than animal or protein-source amino acids. Just be sure you're using the "L-configured" ones; they are identical to the natural food ones and to the kind your body uses efficiently. Do not use D,L-form amino acids; especially do not ever use D,L-methionine as a supplement for an ASD indi-vidual. D,L-mixtures are also manufactured products, and they are intended as animal feed additives. Two common amino acids do not have D or L variants – glycine and taurine, and synthesized forms of these are recommended.

I also endorse use of synthesized mineral supplements as amino acid chelates or amino acid complexes. Synthesized magnesium glycinate has very high bioavailability (efficient uptake from the intestinal tract into the bloodstream). Calcium citrate also has high bio-availability, and its use vastly reduces the lead contamination present in most rock, bone and coral-based supplements. Other essential elements can be purified prior to synthesizing bioavailable complexes as well – zinc, iron, copper, manganese, molybdenum, selenium, iodine and chromium are available as amino acid chelates.

We do not have synthetic forms of essential oils (fatty acids) such as "omega-3" fish oils. The major purity issue with these is mercury content. Cod liver oil (with vitamin A and vitamin D) also is in this category. These supplements can be very helpful to many with ASD, and you should ensure that the ones you use have "less than detectable" mercury content by analytical analysis. Check the label, or perhaps there's a package insert that certifies that the product is "mercury free". "Mercury free" means that, if it's there, it's at a level so low that measuring instruments can't quantify it, or it's at a level that's below the instrument detection limit. If you do not find this information on or with the product, I recommend that you phone, write or email for it, and don't use the product until you're satisfied about it.

Just about all encapsulated or tableted nutritional supplement products necessarily contain ingredients that enable or facilitate economic manufacture, enhance attractiveness to the consumer, or improve utilization once the product has been swallowed. Even dry, powdered charcoal needs some added lubricant to get it into gelatin capsules. I consider flavorings and colorings to be excipients and I don't consider them to be inactive or inert. While flavoring can be a benefit for chewed nutrients, colorings definitely are not. Red, yellow and blue food colorings, the most common ones, can be real troublemakers. Avoid them.

Responsible manufacturers will provide "full disclosure" on the product label – all the ingredients, active and inactive. If the nutritional supplement product doesn't have full disclosure on or in the package, my advice is: don't buy it.

Typical Excipients

- Flavorings – added to free powder products, nutrition bars, chewed wafers, etc.
- Natural flavors extracted from fruits or berries (usually okay)
- Citric acid (usually synthetic) – okay at excipient levels
- Sugars – usually fructose or dextrose, mannitol, xylitol (acceptability depends on amounts)
- Artificial sweeteners – aspartame, sucralose, sorbitol, stevia extract (all can cause problems)
- Lubricants – needed to get powders to flow into capsules or tablet ingredients into the mold
  - Magnesium stearate (okay at excipient levels)
  - Branched-chain amino acids: leucine, sometimes valine (usually okay, but watch amounts for hypoglycemic individuals)
- pH Adjusters – used to control the acid/base feature
  - Adipic acid, citric acid, sodium citrate, bicarbonate (okay)

- Fillers and binders – to fill space so a small amount of active ingredient doesn't get lost or maldistributed, and to hold tablets together. Typical are forms of calcium sulfate, or phosphate, cellulose (plant source usually is best), starches (often cornstarch), maltodextrin (some of these can cause problems)
- Preservatives – because, like it or not, nutrients oxidize or decay with time and with exposure to air.
  - Ascorbate, vitamin E (both ok), sodium benzoate (okay in low amounts, 10-20 mg); BHA, BHT (not okay, avoid), potassium sorbate (okay, discourages mold/yeast).

I expect that your first thought will be, "how do I know this stuff is okay to be taken regularly? Well, you're right, some of it could be of concern, and it's usually a matter of amount.

Citric acid and citrates are generally beneficial because they contribute to cellular energy conversion via the citric acid cycle in cell mitochondria. Also, synthetic citric acid is usually used, and this negates worry about citrus allergies. Natural flavors, however, are just that, so watch out for allergy to strawberry, for example. The sugars usually are necessary for compliance. Often, it's either "tastes okay" or "ugh, no way!" With the typical autistic child, if it tastes bad, it immediately gets spit out onto the floor.

On the topic of lubricants, I'm often asked, "why not use the essential and slippery amino acid leucine for all encapsulated supplement lubrication? Why use mag-stearate?" Well, lubricant contents add up. All the stearate you'd get in 20 typical capsules doesn't amount to what you'd get in a hamburger. But 20 typical capsules could contain a total of 500 to 600 mg of L-leucine. Leucine stimulates the pancreas to release insulin, which lowers blood sugar – not so good for a hypoglycemic person. So, we really don't want to have leucine as the lubricant in all our encapsulated supplements. I'd be worried about more than 200 mg of leucine per day for a hypoglycemic child, and worried about more than 400 mg for a hypoglycemic adult.

pH adjusters are not inert additives. It's just that they don't matter to body physiology when used in the small amounts required for supplement pH balancing. They probably would matter if they were the whole supplement instead of 5% or less of the contents.

On fillers and binders, watch out for cornstarch for those with exquisite corn sensitivity. I've heard of many genuine allergy complaints that turned out to be provoked by cornstarch fillers.

Nowadays, vitamins C or E are often used as preservatives. In doing their job, they get oxidized, just as they do inside our bodies. We either rejuvenate them or dump them. Preservative amounts are relatively tiny and our metabolic capacity for them is adequate. Even the benzoate levels in supplements shouldn't be a problem. Our liver adds glycine (a very plentiful amino acid) to benzoate and the result is hippuric acid, which is dumped in the urine. So, getting rid of benzoate is an easy job for the body provided we're not swamped with it. We can be swamped with benzoate from intestinal dysbiosis, plus soda pop-source amounts. And with autism, the dysbiosis issue isn't trivial, nor is the energy required for detoxication. Adding glycine to benzoate uses one high energy ATP for each benzoate converted to hippurate. No big deal for a few milligrams of benzoate – but don't push it.

The alphabet soup preservatives are mostly bad news – BHA, BHT, TBHQ, etc. BHT, for example, is butylated hydroxytoluene. Why would you eat that?!

NUTRIENT DESCRIPTIONS AND
USE INFORMATION

Doses (Servings)

Strictly speaking, the word "dose" refers to how much medicine should be taken at one time. Nutritional supplements are foods, not medicines. The proper term that corresponds to dose for nutritional supplements is "serving" or 'serving size". That's what you'll find on supplement container labels.

Units and Measures

Supplements come in various forms, such as encapsulated powders or liquids, solid tablets, powders or liquids in plastic bottles or glass jars, and as chewable wafers or bars. Both form and amount cause different units of measurement to be used and posted on labels. To use these nutrients intelligently, and to prevent mistakes, we need to be familiar with the several kinds of measurement units and how they can be converted, one into another.

Metric units of weight are what we encounter most often for supplements – grams, milligrams or micrograms. 1.0 gram(g) = 1000 milligrams (mg) = 1,000,000 micrograms (µg or mcg). Also occasionally encountered is the picogram (pcg) unit. 1000 picograms = 1 microgram.

To put this into perspective, a pound is about 454 g, and one ounce is one-sixteenth of that or about 28 grams. A serving of powdered amino acids, for example, might be measured in grams (3 or 5 g), while a serving of vitamin C usually is measured in milligrams (50 or 100 mg). Some nutrients are needed only in ultratrace amounts, and microgram units then are used. Vitamin B_{12} and folate are examples where the serving amounts could be 10 mcg and 400 mcg respectively.

Sometimes English units (traditional American and British) appear in texts or on products – pounds and ounces. 1 pound = 16 ounces (oz) = 453.6g; 1.0 oz = 28.35g.

These traditional English units are the 'avoirdupois" kind – French for "to have some weight". Why French? Go figure! Ounces avoirdupois are used for commodities of all kinds except: precious metals, gems, powder charges in ammunition, and drugs (medicines). Drugs and the other stuff are measured in units of troy ounces and grains.

1.0 troy ounce = 1.1 avoirdupois ounce

1.0 troy oz = 480 grains (gr); 1.0 gr = 64.8 mg

You probably won't see grains as a unit of measurement on nutritional products, but you may find it on medicines. Apothecaries and pharmacies use grains, and they also may use "drams".

1.0 troy oz = 8 drams = 480 gr; 1.0 dram = 60 gr

Summary:

1.0 gr (troy or apothecary) = 64.8 mg

1.0 dram (apothecary) = 3.89 g; 1.0 dram (avdp) = 1.77g (rarely used)

1.0 oz (avdp) = 28.35 g

1.0 oz (troy) = 31.1 g

What about liquid measures? Here again we have mixed units of measurement – liters, milliliters, pints, fluid ounces, teaspoons, etc. here are some useful relationships that should help.

1 liter (l) = 1000 milliliters (ml) = 1000 cubic centimeters (cc)

1 quart (U.S.) = 32 fluid ounces (oz) = 2 pints = 0.946 l = 946 ml

1 pint = 16 fluid oz = 473 ml

1 fluid oz = 29.5 ml or cc, or approx 30 ml = 2 tablespoons (Tbs or T)

1 Tbs = 15 ml or cc = 3 teaspoons (tsp or t)

1 tsp = 5 ml or cc

A word about three imprecise but often used measures – teaspoons of powder, grams expressed in milliliters and eyedropper drops. Sometimes we are directed to use a teaspoon of a powdered nutrient but we'd like to know how much that is in weight units (grams). For most nutritional supplements, a level [measuring-spoon] teaspoon of powder is about 3 to 4 grams. But this can vary quite a bit because various supplements can be fluffy or dense. If you're uncertain and want to know, call or email the manufacturer to ensure that you're using the intended amount.

For our purposes, 1.0 milliliter (one thousandth of a liter) equals 1.0 cubic centimeter. If the substance occupying that cc or ml is water, then it weighs approximately 1.0 g. If it's a water solution of something – vitamins, mineral salts, amino acids, then it weighs a bit more than 1.0 g, but not much more. Most such water solutions will not weigh more than 1.1 g per ml. For oils, 1.0 ml weighs a little less than 1.0g.

How much fluid is in a drop from an eyedropper? In college, my chemistry professor said 0.05 ml if it's water or an aqueous solution with water-like properties. I did check this by putting 20 drops in a tiny measuring glass and I got just slightly more than 1.0 ml – so 0.05 ml is close enough.

Capsule Sizes

Powdered nutrients are often provided in gelatin capsules, and these come in different sizes. Gelatin capsules are used because they dissolve quickly in the gastrointestinal tract and because binders and other stuff that holds tablets together can be omitted. Another benefit of capsules is that the two halves of the gelatin shell can be pulled apart and the contents added to food or drink for more convenient ingestion.

Six different sizes of capsules are commonly used to hold servings of nutritional supplements. The largest is called double O, denoted OO; the next largest is single O, and then they are numbered 1,2,3 and 4, 4 being the smallest. Usually, small children cannot swallow OO or O-size capsules, and even a number 1 may be a problem. So, before purchasing any encapsulated supplement, take into account –

a) Can my child swallow this size capsule?, or

b) Is it okay to open the capsule and pour the contents onto food to be eaten or into a drink? The answer to this should be available from the supplement supplier/manufacturer.

Capsule Size	Dimensions mm* Length, diameter		Approximate content weight, mg**
OO	23	8.5	600-1100
O	22	7.6	400-850
1	19	6.9	350-600
2	18	6.4	250-450
3	16	5.8	200-375
4	14	5.3	150-280

* mm = millimeters; 1.0 inch = 25.4 mm

** Approximate because different powdered nutrients have different densities and packing   characteristics. Some are heavy crystals; some are fluffy and flake-like.

Alpha-Ketoglutaric Acid

Alpha-ketoglutaric acid (or "alpha-ketoglutarate") is an extremely important organic acid needed for nitrogen balance, especially in the brain and CNS. It is also a critical component of energy conversion in cell mitochondria, and it is part of the mitochondrial antioxidant mechanism.

Indications of Need

A diagnosis of or signs consistent with: ammonia excess, hyperammonemia, blood nitrogen or nitrogen compound excess; exposure to excesses of arsenic, mercury, lead or antimony; exposure to xenobiotic chemicals (pesticides, herbicides, fungicides, anesthetics, petrochemicals, combustion fumes/smoke, nitriles or cyanide); stool too basic (pH too high – ammonia from dysbiosis); diagnosis of mitochondrial disorder, oxidant stress.

When and How Much?

This depends on the problem and the reason for its use. Alpha-ketoglutaric acid does not stop excessive formation of ammonia , rather, it extends cell and tissue abilities to cope with ammonia. It chemically combines with ammonia to form glutamic acid – a much less toxic substance than ammonia. If ammonia excess is the problem, gram quantities per day of alpha-ketoglutarate (buffered) can be beneficial – 50 to 200 mg per Kg body weight. A taurine supplement might help further by encouraging the conversion of glutamic acid to glutamine. Lesser amounts of alpha-ketoglutaric acid, 25 to 100 mg/kg may be helpful for other problems. Usually, this nutrient is available in capsules of 300 milligrams buffered to prevent acidity. Divided doses with meals works best; do not use unbuffered alpha-ketoglutaric acid.

Adverse Response to Alpha-Ketoglutaric Acid.

Since the beginnings of its use as a nutritional product in the early 1980s, there have been no reports of problems that I know of, with two exceptions. The first was a teenager who took a whole 100-capsule bottle of 300 mg capsules in one day. That's 30 grams. He exhibited hyperactivity for the next 24 hours but had no other symptoms. The second was nausea traced to poor product quality. During manufacturing, storage and use, alpha-ketoglutaric acid should be kept dry with the bottle tightly closed. If the product is dark colored (instead of a white powder), or if it smells bad (fishy or foul), do not use it.

About Alpha-Ketoglutaric Acid (Optional Reading)

In the 1980s, our son was diagnosed as having elevated ammonia in blood but without a problem in urea formation and without evident dysbiosis. Something in his metabolism wasn't going right, and the two doctors in charge were baffled. We followed instructions and lowered his dietary protein intake, and I decided to investigate further. I hit the books, and an interesting find came from Albert Lehninger's famed textbook, <u>Biochemistry</u>. Dr. Lehninger was a professor of medicine at Johns Hopkins University. The find was that the body has its own remedy for ammonia besides the liver's urea cycle. In fact, in the brain and central nervous system, this remedy is the major pathway of ammonia disposal. Here's how it works –

In the brain, some alpha-ketoglutaric acid combines with ammonia to make glutamic acid. This is what's supposed to happen. The brain doesn't have direct access to a urea-forming cycle as the liver does. So the brain needs a fast, efficient alternative. After the glutamic acid is made, we still have a problem. Glutamic acid is very slow to cross the brain-blood barrier, it's an excitatory neurotransmitter, and too much of it causes trouble. To counter that problem, the brain has a second step to its ammonia detoxication process. It adds another ammonia (as an "amide") to glutamic acid. That changes it into glutamine. This is the step that taurine promotes.

Glutamine, with its ammonia load aboard, readily passes out of the brain. Via blood, it goes to the kidneys for excretion, or it's disassembled and the resulting ammonia is changed into urea in the liver.

So, my problem was to come up with some alpha-ketoglutaric acid. It was not available anywhere as a nutritional supplement (~1980). It was available as a specialty chemical; it is a natural, big-time biochemical in our bodies, but its use in humans seemed to only be in clinical research studies. Nobody would make the jump from research uses to nutritional supplement use.

It took over a year, but finally someone came along who could help – Mr. Jim Dews. Jim operated a nutritional supplement company in Texas, and he custom-made various nutritional products for doctors. We put our heads together; he came up with a buffering formulation, and then made a pilot batch. He and I took several capsules without ill effect. My family, Dews' employees, and some of Dr. Philpott's staff in Oklahoma City also tried it. In the 1980s, Dr. Philpott was one of our son's physicians. Eventually, since it was a natural biochemical in the body, he selected some patients to try it. In most cases, the feedback was – Wow! Where'd this extra energy come from!

Lab tests followed, showing that blood ammonia levels are lowered by alpha-ketoglutaric acid supplements. In fact, normal alpha-ketoglutaric acid levels become abnormally low when ammonia is elevated. There even was a contemporary article from the New England Journal of Medicine showing exactly this for individuals with a metabolic fault to the urea cycle – Batshaw ML, Roan Y et al. "Cerebral Dysfunction in Asymptomatic Carriers of Ornithine Transcarbamylase Deficiency", *NEJ Med* 302 no.9 (Feb 28, 1980) 482-85; see Fig 4, p 484.

So, giving alpha-ketoglutaric acid pretty much has to work as a nutritional strategy for elevated ammonia. We didn't try to patent alpha-ketoglutarate. After Jim Dews had it exclusively for about two years, I got Klaire Labs to manufacture it, too. After that, it grew on its own.

Inside cells there are several chemical processes that make and use alpha-ketoglutaric acid. One such process inside cell mitochondria is called the "citric acid cycle" – it's an energy conversion, acid-base-balancing and coenzyme-activating mechanism. Another process is called the "malate shuttle". In that one, alpha-ketoglutarate travels out of the mitochondria, goes through hydrogen addition and goes back in as malic acid. That's a major process for antioxidant protection (hydrogen delivery) for mitochondria.

Inside mitochondria, in the citric acid cycle, alpha-ketoglutaric acid and coenzyme A are changed into succinyl-coenzyme A by an enzyme complex that also forms activated niacin coenzyme, NADH, as well as CO_2 (for bicarbonate). The succinyl CoA, by the way, is what vitamin B_{12} as adenosylcobalamin assists in making from methylmalonyl-CoA

(MMA-CoA); methylmalonic acid comes from propionic acid. See Vitamin chapter, B_{12} section. So, the mitochondrial chemistry of alpha-ketoglutaric acid, vitamin B_{12} and carnitine are all closely related.

Literature – Alpha-Ketoglutaric Acid

Lehninger A, Biochemistry, Worth Publishers, various editions 1970s, descriptions of functions of alpha-ketoglutarate: amino transfer, ammonia complexing, malate shuttle, citric acid cycle participant, etc.

Batshaw M et al. "Cerebral Dysfunction in Asymptomatic Carriers of Ornithine Transcarbamylase Deficiency" N.E.J.Med 302(9), Feb 28, 1980 482-85. Shows clinical data on depletion of alpha-ketoglutarate with ammonia elevation.

Moore SJ et al. "Efficacy of α-ketoglutaric Acid in the Antagonism of Cyanide Intoxication" Toxicol and Appl Pharmacol 82 (1986) 40-44.

Harpers Biochemistry, Lange Medical Publications, multiple editions – descriptions of what alpha-ketoglutarate does physiologically.

Amino Acids (except Taurine)

When humans eat animal or vegetable proteins, our digestive processes are supposed to break these proteins apart to form the small molecules that are the building units of our protein. These building units are the molecules we call amino acids. "Amino" derives from the ammonia-like pieces of the molecule (a nitrogen atom plus two hydrogen atoms = "amino"). The acid part makes the molecule reactive and able to combine readily with other amino acids.

The objective of digestion is to provide a pool of free-form amino acids that can be reassembled inside our organs and tissues in specific sequences to make human proteins, peptides and some very specialized products. Among the specialized products formed from one or more amino acids are: creatine, serotonin, melatonin, adrenal catecholamines, glutathione, melanins (biochemicals that give color to tissue), porphyrins, and purines and pyrimidines, and nucleotides. Nucleotides are molecules that participate in cellular growth, replication, and information processing. Amino acids also are used to construct enzymes, antibodies, immunoglobulins and hormones, and they help to operate detoxication chemistry. Amino acids combine with or conjugate toxic substances; they get rid of excess nitrogen as urea, and they form bile salts from cholesterol using the amino acids glycine or taurine. Bile and urine are the two major fluids that carry toxicants out of the body.

Indications of Need

Unfortunately, amino acid adequacy is so necessary to health that a detailed list of deficiency symptoms isn't practical, especially when we account for the fact that at least eight are are essential for life (nine counting histidine)! An analytical measure of need for specific amino acids is a quantitative amino acid analysis of fasting blood plasma or of non-fasting 24-hour urine. Spot analyses of urine ratioed to creatinine are less desirable and can be problematic in autism/ASD. (See chapter on creatine.) Spot blood plasma analysis (non-fasting) is only useful if the laboratory's reference range and food intake parameters apply – most clinical laboratories do not accommodate requests for non-fasting blood amino acid analysis. This is an area of diagnosis and intervention where a professional nutritionist or your doctor can be of help. You will need a doctor to order an amino acid test, and the doctor or nutritionist or the laboratory's professional staff should be of help in explaining test results.

An individual who shows benefit from digestive enzyme use might benefit from an amino acid supplement, as might one whose diet is low in protein foods. Chronic problems with detoxication, inflammation, immune or neurological functions might benefit from amino acid supplements.

There are balanced blends of essential and protein-forming amino acids that can be used on a trial basis, and that you can order from nutritional suppliers. Such blends are generally safe to use in amounts suggested by the manufacturer or by your doctor/nutritionist. I formulated a blend based on amino acid measurements from autistic children; I'll tell you about that one in a following section of this chapter. Just be aware that success with a moderate amount does not mean that doubling the amount will be twice as good.

There are a several disease conditions that contraindicate amino acid use. Except for hyperammonemia, these are rare in ASD. Hyperammonemia, elevated ammonia in blood, can be a serious condition that requires medical advice and possibly special interventions. A simple blood test at a local hospital tells the tale; accurate ammonia testing has to be done very promptly (not with sent-in specimens). Lowering dietary protein, eliminating infections and dysbiotic gut flora, and oral use of alpha-ketoglutaric acid are nutritional strategies for reducing ammonia levels. Please see "Adverse Responses to Amino Acid Supplements" in this chapter for further contraindications to supplementing amino acids.

When and How Much?

With autism or ASD, my advice is: never begin nutritional intervention with amino acid supplements, except for taurine. An amino acid supplement is a Tier 5 item. The "when" for amino acids is after intestinal and digestive problems have been addressed and after you've decided on a special diet, if one is beneficial. Why is this? Because some of the amino acids could wind up being misused by dysbiotic flora. Also, a special diet can result in big changes in need for nutritional supplements.

I really don't want to scare you away from an eventual trial of an amino acid supplement, but I've been asked so many times, "What could go wrong?" Here's some of it.

Cystine, cysteine and N-acetylcysteine (NAC) are culture media for the Candida genus of yeast. Also, cystine or cysteine or NAC supplementation can mobilize toxicants (such as mercury) from sequestered sites inside cells. But this mobilization will not necessarily lead to detoxication and may worsen the extent of the contamination. Wait until the gastrointestinal tract is healthy and functional, and wait until metabolism is improved, especially that of glutathione, and wait until some of the oxidant stress and inflammation are alleviated.

Glutamine, when malabsorbed and chewed on by dysbiotic bacterial flora, produces succinic acid. Most elevations of succinic acid found by organic acid analysis of the urine of autistics come from glutamine; levels resolve when the digestive function is normalized. Succinic acid can have toxic effects when it's not in the cellular compartments where it is supposed to be.

Clostridia ingesting phenylalanine, tyrosine and tryptophan produce phenol, para-cresol, phenylpropionic acid, and hydroxyphenylpropionic acid (HPPA) which, when hydroxylated in the liver, becomes the dihydroxyl form, DHPPA. DHPPA is what William Shaw found in the urine of autistics years ago. That and similar compounds are markers for dysbiotic gut flora offered by Great Plains Laboratory of Lenexa, KS, MetaMetrix Laboratory of Norcross GA, and Genova Diagnostics of Asheville NC. From these same amino acids, Clostridia also produce other substances of varying toxicities: phenylacetic acid, phenyllactic acid, indole and indoleacetic acid.

Tryptophan, when it is consumed by some intestinal bacteria (instead of being absorbed into blood) can also be changed into another form of propionic acid (indolylpropionate), which, after absorption into body tissue, is changed into indolylacrylic acid. Forms of acrylic acid are real bad guys; they destroy fatty acid (cell) membranes. The liver tries to detoxify the indolylacrylic acid by attaching the amino acid glycine to its reactive part. The result is indolylacryloylglycine or "IAG". IAG is what Paul Shattock's team found in the urine of autistics years ago, and it was turned into a laboratory test marker. The test is offered by Genova Diagnostics of Asheville NC. When elevated, it indicates: malabsorption of tryptophan, probable intestinal dysbiosis, and increased detoxication load on the liver.

So, parents and doctors, there are two lab tests (DHPPA, IAG) that you can do to see if amino acids are being misused due to malabsorption plus intestinal dysbiosis. My experience is that both often increase a bit in urine with amino acid supplements. If initial levels are very high, then you've got work to do before using amino acid supplements. If initial levels are normal and go up by 50% - honestly, that's not bad and attributable symptoms are unlikely (but symptoms tell the tale, not test results). However, if IAG or DHPPA levels double, triple, or go even higher, then you've got dysbiosis to clean up before using amino acid supplements.

Supplementing Amino Acids Per Test Results

The most accurate way to learn which amino acids are needed for an individual, and how much, is to do an amino acid analysis. Before you do this, find out if the laboratory provides a supplement schedule, when appropriate, with the results. If an amino acid report does not have a supplement schedule, you will need to consult a professional nutritionist for guidance about supplementation.

I'm partial to 24-hour urine because it tells a 24-hour tale. Plasma is okay, but it is a fasting test which is a snapshot in time of what's circulating in the blood. Urine shows what's left over after a whole day's activities. If there's too little left over, then more is needed. When urine is used to judge amino acid status, renal clearance should also be judged as okay by your doctor. He or she can assess this from a simple blood chemistry test. I strongly advise not ratioing 24-hour urine or spot urine analyte levels to creatinine for autistic individuals. The supplement schedule from a lab report can be filled by a compounding pharmacy upon receiving a doctor's prescription appended to the supplement schedule page. Some compounding pharmacies are:

- Apothecary, Bethesda MD, 800-869-9160, fax 301-493-4671
- ApotheCure, Dallas TX, 800-969-6601, fax 800-687-5252
- College Pharmacy, Colorado Springs CO, 800-888-9358-, fax 800-556-5893

- Creative Compounds, Wilsonville OR, 877-585-6111, fax 503-570-2831
- Falls Pharmacy, Snoqualmie, WA, 877-392-7948, fax 425-888-6870
- Hopewell Pharmacy, Hopewell NJ, 800-792-6670, fax 800-417-3864
- Key Pharmacy, Kent, WA, 800-878-1322, fax 206-878-1114
- Lee Silsby Pharmacy, Cleveland OH, 800-918-8831, fax 216-321-4303
- University Pharmacy, Troy MI, 248-267-5002, fax 248-267-5003
- Wellness, Birmingham AL:, 800-227-2627, fax 205-369-0302

There's one complication that I've frequently had to contend with on amino acid lab tests. It's taurine. Ninety-nine percent of the time, high urine taurine means urinary wasting of taurine (see chapter on taurine). High plasma taurine is an occasional finding in autism/ASD, and it's consistent with inflammation, increased immune defense and possible cell breakage, or oxidant or tissue damage. Taurine concentration inside cells is generally much higher than normal blood plasma levels.

The Amino Acid Supplement I Formulated

In 2001, I did a survey of over 60 urine amino acid analyses on autistic children, ages 3-9. These kids (47 males, 14 females) had gone through diet trials, and many were on special diets. They had been treated with antifungals and antibacterials and were on probiotics supplements. However, only a few were reported to be on digestive enzymes, which definitely help protein digestion and amino acid adequacy. Here's what I found.

Amino acid judged to be nutritionally low or lower	% of 61 ASD children
Taurine	62
Lysine	59
Phenylalanine	54
Methionine	51
Tyrosine	38
Leucine	36
Glutamine	33
Valine	30
Tryptophan	28
Asparagine	26
Arginine	25
Isoleucine	23

Cyst(e)ine is excluded because urine isn't a good specimen for assessing its adequacy. For taurine, both low and high with wasting-pattern consorts (beta-alanine, beta-aminoisobutyric) count as low. "Low" is below one standard deviation below the mean of the normal range, i.e., nutritional low and lower (not necessarily a below-reference-range deficiency).

These nutritional subnormalities tabulated above may have resulted from the special diets, or they may have persisted since before intervention. Pretreatment analyses often show as many or even more marginal or low levels. Remember, changing the diet and killing bad flora are cleanup procedures. They don't necessarily repair digestive dysfunctions that might have been preexisting conditions, and they don't ensure nutritional adequacy.

A unique blend that is designed to compensate for the suboptimal levels as tallied above is available from Kirkman Laboratories of Lake Oswego, OR, 1-800-245-8282, "Amino Support". (I receive no compensation for sale of this product and no compensation of any kind from Kirkman Labs.)

The essential amino acid tryptophan is not included in "Amino Support". This amino acid is especially contraindicated as a supplement when intestinal dysbiosis is present, particularly in ASD. It is my opinion that analytic evidence of normal intestinal function and flora are prerequisites to use of oral tryptophan supplements. When there is malabsorption, as mentioned previously, this amino acid is what certain bacteria use to make IAG (indolylacrylglycine).

Other blends of essential and protein amino acids are available OTC and from other nutritional supplement companies. For children 5 to 12 years of age, 3 to 9 grams per day of an amino acid blend can be beneficial; younger children should be given lesser amounts. Teens and adults may need 5 to 12 grams/day. Use of any single amino acid other than taurine should be done only under the guidance of a health professional.

Adverse Responses to Amino Acid Supplements?

With adverse responses, the first concern should be: is gut dysbiosis still present? Most often, that's the problem. I advise taking natural, herbal-type antibacterial, antifungal/anti-yeast supplements when dysbiosis is suspected. I strongly advise continued use of antifungal/anti-yeast herbals if and when oral cystine, N-acetylcysteine (NAC), glutathione, or lipoic acid are used.

The next concern is rapid transit in the gastrointestinal tract, which may be coincident with diarrhea or runny stools. If that's not caused by dysbiosis, then it's usually intolerance or reactivity to a food or medication. The problem is that the fast transit may be allowing the amino acids to reach to large bowel (where lots of bacteria reside). If that's going on, then don't give amino acid supplements. Ditto for the opposite case, constipation. Even normal gut flora can misbehave when presented with food they shouldn't have.

Ensure that there is B-vitamin adequacy and also adequate supplements of minerals, especially magnesium and zinc. These are needed for metabolism of amino acids.

Health professionals are cautioned that some unusual metabolic conditions are contraindications for amino acid supplementation. Some of these are as follows.

- Hyperammonemia – no amino acids until the condition is completely understood, then maybe none, or only selected ones – this is not uncommon with ASD.
- Renal failure (poor kidney clearance); do not give amino acids if this is the case.
- Histidinemia – avoid histidine
- Cystinuria – avoid cysteine, cysteine, NAC, and limit glutathione; measure blood plasma for status of lysine, arginine and ornithine. Antioxidant nutrients may be beneficial.
- Lysinuric intolerance – avoid lysine
- Hartnup syndrome – avoid tryptophan
- Hyperphenylalaninuria – avoid phenylalanine; determine if tyrosine is needed.
- Tyrosinemia – avoid tyrosine

- Branched-chain amino acid excesses – avoid leucine, isoleucine and valine, at least until the biochemical reasons are understood.
- If SAM is being supplemented (which I do <u>not</u> advise), expect limited tolerance for methionine.
- Carnitine deficiency
- Vitamin B deficiency

About Amino Acids (Optional Reading)

Obviously, when digestion goes wrong, the body supply of amino acids can run short, and the processes that depend upon them can go wrong as well. My experience is that protein maldigestion can be quite accurately assessed by amino acid analysis. Test results showing decreased essentials and elevated dietary peptides (usually, anserine and carnosine in urine) are analytical evidence of incomplete digestive proteolysis – maldigestion. With malabsorption, some of the needed dietary nutrients, including amino acids, are carried to the large intestine and may be lost in the stool. Malabsorption is suggested by low urine or blood threonine, together with other low essentials, while the dietary peptides may be within normal limits. Threonine is an essential amino acid and is the slowest one to cross from the lumen of the small intestine into the portal blood.

The nutritionally essential amino acids are:

Leucine, Isoleucine and Valine

These are "branched-chain" essential amino acids needed for collagen tissue formation. They are called 'branched-chain' because the carbon chain in each one is forked or branched. Assimilation of these is quite dependent upon pancreatic and mucosal peptidase enzymes that work in the small intestine. In autism, levels of leucine, isoleucine and valine may be low if peptidase function is weak. Deficient levels of leucine, isoleucine and/or valine are not typical in autism, but nutritionally-low levels (one standard deviation below mean of normal) seem to occur in about one in four or five autistics per urine amino acid analysis.

Methionine

This one is the king of essentials. It brings sulfur and methyl groups into the body, participates in methylation after it's transformed into "SAM", and is the essential precursor of cysteine and taurine. Methionine assimilation is somewhat dependent upon adequate stomach acid and pepsinogen becoming pepsin. Insufficient stomach acidity and inadequate pepsin are not reported to be common in autism. Yet, prior to interventions, methionine is on the low side in about half of autistic children, per blood plasma analysis. This is ascribed to deficient recycling of homocysteine back to methionine via the methionine synthase enzyme complex.

Phenylalanine

This amino acid is the precursor of tyrosine, which forms the adrenal catecholamines and the part of thyroglobulin to which iodine attaches to make thyroid hormones. Phenylalanine is low in some autistic children. However, it is high in PKU or phenylketonuria, which may feature autism. PKU is rarely found now as an untreated condition.

Tryptophan

This one is used in the body to make serotonin and melatonin, and a little bit of it even becomes niacin, vitamin B_3. Tryptophan can be low in blood in some autistics if maldigestion or malabsorption occurs. In such cases, tryptophan can be changed into indolylpropionic acid by gut bacteria. As mentioned previously, this leads to the IAG found frequently in the urine of ASD individuals having malabsorption and possibly intestinal dysbiosis as well. Occasionally, tryptophan is used to form large amounts of serotonin in abdominal tissues, and the availability of tryptophan (to become serotonin) may then be limited in the CNS. Serotonin produced in abdominal tissues acts as a vasoconstrictor. It decreases capillary blood flow in the intestinal mucosa and restricts uptake of toxins (from dysbiosis) or peptides and undigested parts of food. Elevated blood serotonin has been reported to occur in about 25% of autistics in numerous studies beginning in the 1960s through to the present.

If serotonin is low in the CNS, consequences include low melatonin, poor sleep patterns, and increased sensitivity to light and sound.

Lysine

This essential amino acid is a major component of muscle protein. It is the link point in aminotransferase enzymes ("transaminases") between the enzyme and the coenzyme, pyridoxal 5-phosphate. Lysine is commonly deficient in autistics before dietary intervention. In protein, lysine is the target sought after by homocysteine thiolactone. This is homocysteine that got hijacked because the paraoxonase enzyme wasn't able to rescue it, possibly following exposure to organophosphate spray of some sort. Please refer back to the part on organophosphate toxicants in the Background chapter.

Threonine

This one is the essential precursor of serine and glycine. It is one of the few amino acids that allow glycoprotein formation – attachment of a carbohydrate or sugar to a protein. Cell membranes contain glycoproteins as do blood group substances, the compounds that make blood types different. Immunoglobulins, interferon, and cell-cell recognition substances include glycoproteins. These structures are essential for proper immune function. Blood or urine threonine is often low in medically defined malabsorption syndromes, but it is only occasionally found to be low in autism.

Histidine

Before about 1985, this amino acid was considered to be essential only for infants. It is now considered to be essential for adults as well, and it's what is used to make the hormone histamine in our tissues. Histidine is usually provided by a dietary dipeptide that is digested either in the small intestine or internally – carnosine. Anserine, a sister peptide, contains methylated histidine, and we may or may not derive histidine from that source. Histidine is very important in autism. Some of it is processed to form "FIGlu" (formiminoglutamic acid). FIGlu combines with tetrahydrofolate to make 5-formimino-tetrahydrofolate. This is eventually changed into folate forms that are needed for purine synthesis (adenosine, for example). An uncommon disease condition, histidinemia (with too much histidine) can feature autistic-like traits. Nutrients that are important for histidine metabolism include folic acid, vitamins B_6 and B_{12}, and zinc.

Cysteine

May be considered a nonessential or conditionally essential amino acid because much of the need can be supplied by methionine. By my own estimates, about 50 to 65% of cysteine normally comes from methionine. The remainder is from direct dietary sources (cysteine + cystine + related other forms). Cysteine is the rate-limiting amino acid for formation of glutathione; it contributes significantly (depending on diet) to taurine synthesis, and it is the major source of sulfate for sulfation. Cysteine is low/deficient, per blood analysis, in many autistics. Special collection and laboratory procedures are needed to accurately quantify its level in blood plasma or serum. It is not accurately measured by HPLC amino acid analysis of "sent in" blood samples. Oral supplementation of this amino acid is unsafe and is not advised.

Arginine

This "semiessential" amino acid is made in liver tissue as part of the "urea cycle", a sequence of chemical changes that detoxifies ammonia by changing it into urea. The problem is, it's needed elsewhere and the urea cycle mostly uses what it makes. So, we need a dietary source, too. The semiessential classification means we make it but not enough. A very major use of arginine is synthesis of creatine (please see creatine chapter). Another use is formation of nitric oxide, a chemical messenger that's involved in regulation of many physiological processes such as vascular tone, blood pressure, muscle action and inflammatory response.

Literature – Amino Acids

Harper's Biochemistry (any available edition), Lange Publishers
Chaitow L Amino Acids in Therapy, Healing Arts Press, Rochester VT (1988)
Recommended Dietary Allowances 10th Ed., National Research Council, Food and Nutrition, Board, National Academy Press, Washington DC (1989) Chapter 6, p 52-77.
Bremer HJ, Duran M et al. Disturbances of Amino Acid Metabolism: Clinical Chemistry and Diagnosis Urban & Schwarzenberg (1981) 270-274.
Jepson JB "Hartnup Disease" Chapter 66 in Stanbury J et al. The Metabolic Basis of Inherited Disease 4th ed.McGraw-Hill (1978) 1566-68
Elsden SR, Hilton MG and Waller JM "The end products of the metabolism of aromatic amino acids by Clostridia" Arch Microbiol 107 no.3 (1976) 283-88.

L-Carnitine

Carnitine is a transporter molecule made inside the cells of our body. It also can be supplemented quite effectively and goes to the cellular area where it is needed. That area is the inner mitochondrial membrane (see glossary) where carnitine transports long-chain fats (as acylcarnitine) into the mitochondrial compartment. Here, the processed fat is oxidized and utilized to form carbon dioxide and bicarbonate, water, chemically active cofactors (NADH), and the body's high-energy dynamo molecule, adenosine triphosphate, ATP. Brain ATP, by the way, has been measured (scanned) to be subnormal in autism by Dr. Nancy Minshew, et al., *Biol.Psychiatry* 33 (1993) 762-73.

Indications of Need

In my opinion, a diagnosis of autism is sufficient to warrant trial use of L-carnitine supplements. Specific findings consistent with carnitine need include: (1) blood carnitine deficiency or abnormal levels of various carnitine-associated metabolites; (2) any analytical results indicating methylation deficits (vitamin B_{12} or folate disorders, elevated urine FIGlu, homocysteine deficiency or excess, adenosine excess); (3) benefit from supplements that involve methylation (melatonin, DMG, TMG); (4) abnormal levels of mitochondrial distress markers (blood pyruvate or lactate excess, high alanine/lysine ratio in blood, elevated blood ammonia, abnormal urine/blood levels of citric acid cycle components, excess urine/blood adipic and /or suberic acid); (5) exposure to or excesses of chemicals/biochemicals that carnitine removes from mitochondria (valproic acid and 3-to-8 carbon chain fatty acids, propionic to octanoic, including methylglutaric); (6) chronic fatigue, limited endurance, muscle weakness; (7) exposure to (toxic) xenobiotics or chemicals that may induce renal wasting(8) recent or frequent use of antibiotic medications. Immediately after birth, the infant shifts toward more fatty acids and less glucose for cellular energy requirements. If autism or ASD is considered to be a risk for the infant, then seek medical advice about supplementing L-carnitine early on.

When and How Much?

First of all, never, never use D,L-carnitine. I don't think any of this is still on the market as it was in health food stores in the 1980s. But with foreign supply sources coming into increasing use, ensure that what you use is only L-configured carnitine. D-carnitine blocks what L-carnitine is supposed to do. Moms, if you're expecting, and if there's a known risk of ASD in the family, then consult your doctor about possible supplementation of L-carnitine during pregnancy. Some infant formulas contain L-carnitine, but amounts may be insufficient. Supplemental carnitine is often provided in the more stable form, acetyl-L-carnitine, and this is an excellent form to use.

The amount that is appropriate for an individual infant or child may be a decision for your healthcare professional. My experience is that quite a bit is needed to have benefit, but start low and go up gradually with the supplemental amounts. A two year old may require 250 mg twice a day, and a five year old may benefit from 500 mg twice a day. Adults may need even more.

A guideline from the pharmacy handbook, <u>Drug Facts and Comparisons</u>, is 50 milligrams per kilogram of body weight per day. So, for a 25 lb. child, that would be about 570 mg/d, and for a 50 lb child, about 1140 mg/d. More than that is often needed and beneficial, but should be at the discretion of a physician. Acetyl-L-carnitine goes well with meals, and gelatin capsules of it (usually 250 mg amounts) can be opened and the power sprinkled on prepared food or dissolved in drinks – it is water soluble. Acetyl-L-carnitine has a slightly sour-to-bitter taste, so sweetening may make it more palatable, or it's usually unnoticed if it's put in orange or grapefruit juice.

Adverse Response to L-Carnitine

As above, ensure that the supplement is L-carnitine or acetyl-L-carnitine and not D,L-carnitine. If this supplement is started at high amounts, above 50 mg/kg body wt/

day, some will experience transient nausea and perhaps diarrhea. <u>Facts and Comparisons</u> reports additional problems of cramps and vomiting. For some, it may be necessary to start at 25 mg/kg/day. These symptoms should disappear within 24 hours of discontinuance. <u>Facts and Comparisons</u> adds that there is no lasting toxicity reported from overdosing.

About L-Carnitine (Optional Reading)

In the cells of our body, formation of carnitine starts with lysine, that which is attached to other amino acids in peptide or protein forms. At the very start, a theoretical concern could be with the "pitfall" form of homocysteine (homocysteine thiolactone), which may accumulate if the enzyme paraoxonase is inhibited or genetically weak. Biochemical research indicates that homocysteine thiolactone binds to lysine in peptides and proteins and prevents it from participating in metabolism.

The first step in synthesis is methylation of the lysine by S-adenosylmethionine, "SAM", and this has to occur three times in succession to make tri-methyl-lysine (TML). Here, I have real concerns for the 20-30% of ASD children with hard evidence of impaired SAM methylation. Clinical studies of this have been published by Drs. Stubbs, James, and others. To progress to the next step, trimethyllysine needs alpha-ketoglutarate (A-Kg) and ascorbate (vitamin C). Deficiencies of these can lead to more problems. The next step requires vitamin B_6 as pyridoxal 5'-phosphate (P5P). At this point, those of you who are experienced in the nutritional needs of autistic people are no doubt wondering if there's any carnitine at all being made in some of these individuals.

Eventually, after even more ascorbate and alpha-ketoglutarate are used, we've made L-carnitine.

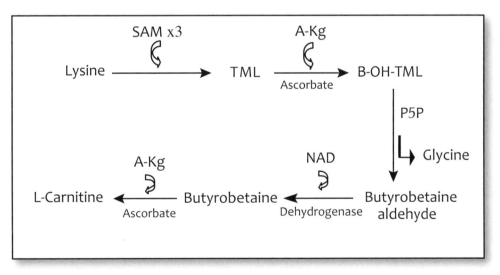

So, has carnitine adequacy been measured in autism? Yes. Is it adequate? No, it's not! – Filipek et al. *J.Autism Dev.Disord* <u>34</u>(6), Dec 2004, 615-623. Eighty three percent of those tested had free and total carnitine levels below the laboratory reference mean. Thirty six percent had total carnitine at levels less than one-standard deviation below the mean. Two authoritative reference laboratories were used: Mayo and Associated Regional and University Pathologists (ARUP). The 83% and 37% results are averages of both labs' findings; ARUP tested 39 males and 15 females while Mayo tested 38 males and 8 females.

Carnitine has also been studied by Dr. MacFabe as part of the propionate/rodent autism model at the U of Western Ontario. Dr. MacFabe's team reports altered levels of carnitine-fatty acid compounds following exposure to short-chain fatty acids. This is coincident with induced ASD-like behaviors in animals. Thomas RH et al., "Altered brain phospholipid and acylcarnitine profiles in propionic acid infused rodents: further development of a potential model of autism spectrum disorders". *J. Neurochem* 2010 Apr; 113(2):515-29.

During the period 2002-2009, a number of scientific papers reported studies on carnitine transporters – biochemical systems that help carnitine find its way intra- and extracellularly. These transporters occur throughout the body, including in brain tissue and in the blood-brain barrier. Defects in these transporters now are described and add another dimension to carnitine deficiency problems. Some carnitine transporters are multi-functional with respect to what they can escort in and out of body tissue. Dr. Ingrid Tien, Hospital for Sick Children, Toronto, published research that calls into question the ability to properly handle some antibiotics (cephalosporins), and the calcium-channel blocker verapamil, as well as valproate and chemicals and drugs, when multi-functional transporters (OCTN1, OCTN2) are defective. See Tien I, "Carnitine transport: pathophysiology and metabolism of known molecular defects" *J.Inherit Metab Dis* 26(2-3), 2003, 147-169.

Carnitine transporter defect is an example of a metabolic fault that can potentially cause both a detoxication deficiency and autistic traits, and I wouldn't be too quick to blame it on genetics. Check out the publication by Pochini cited below in Literature – Carnitine. Many transporters have the "sticky" amino acid cysteine at their active site. It grabs onto what's to be transported. Well, just about anything from mercury to some big foreign chemical can clog up the works if it sticks to cysteine. Often, it takes glutathione to clean up such clogs. It's too bad the individual with ASD often is short on that too.

Literature – Carnitine

Broquist H " Carnitine", Chapt 29 in Shils et al. <u>Modern Nutrition in Health and Disease</u>, 8th ed, Lea & Febiger 1994

Rebouche C "Carnitine metabolism and human nutrition" *J. Applied Nutr* 10(2) 1988 99-111

Pliophys A and Kasricka I "L-Carnitine as a treatment for Rett syndrome" *Southern Med J* 86(12) 1993 1411-12

Pochini L et al. "Inactivation by omeprazole of the carnitine transporter (OCTN2) reconstituted in liposomes" *Chem.Biol. Interact* 179(2-3) 2009 394-401.

Carnosine

Composed of two amino acids, carnosine is a natural dietary substance that comes primarily from dietary meat and fish. A small amount is thought to be made internally. Over the years it has been used nutritionally and therapeutically for enhancement of muscle mass and alleviation of muscular dystrophy. Recently, carnosine has been used clinically, with some success, in alleviating autistic traits in some ASD children, especially those with seizure conditions.

Indications of Need

Per parent reports, indications for possible benefit are seizures or seizure-like episodes and difficulty with improving socialization and verbal communication skills. To this I add the condition that carnosine not be excessive per plasma or urine amino acid analysis. Histidine deficiency (per amino acid analysis) could be an indication of benefit from carnosine supplementation.

When and How Much?

Carnosine usually is packaged in gelatin capsules, in 200 milligram amounts. Parent reports to me have been that young children 3 to 5 years of age may benefit from 2 to 3 capsules/day (400 to 600 mg). Older children 6 to 12 years of age may need 3 to 6 capsules/day (600 to 1200 mg). Start with one capsule and increase gradually with this supplement, because adverse effects are possible and I've gotten reports of help at first followed by relapse.

Adverse Responses to Carnosine

Carnosine is a dipeptide – two amino acids linked together – histidine and beta-alanine. Too much of either of these can cause problems when –

- Histidinemia/uria is present (too much histidine)
- Urinary taurine wasting is occurring, often because beta-alanine already is high
- Taurine in blood/cells is below normal levels
- There's a true copper excess/zinc insufficiency in cells or tissues
- Creatine is deficient per blood assay.

Some of these problems may be correctable such that carnosine supplementation can be continued or tried later. Increasing the daily taurine supplement by up to 50% may help if the issue is low or insufficient taurine. You need blood and urine amino acid analyses to gauge this.

If your child is one of the unusual ones with histidinemia, forget carnosine.

Use of carnosine when there is a creatine deficit is very problematic, and it may be best to wait until creatine is addressed (Tier 5). The problem here is interference by beta-alanine with a creatine synthesis step (making guanidinoacetate). This has only been reported to me twice, but if seizures get worse with carnosine use, stop immediately and ask for a blood measurement of creatine. If it's low, work on that (see chapter on Creatine.)

About Carnosine (Optional Reading)

Noting the beneficial effects ascribed to homocarnosine, a neurotransmitter made in humans, Dr. Michael Chez et al. tried therapeutic use of L-carnosine on a group of autistic children in a placebo-controlled study. They reported improvements in socialization, communication and behavior. (See Literature-Carnosine.) When I questioned Dr. Chez about the types of autistic individuals that he had most success with, using carnosine, he replied that the individuals with seizures showed the most significant benefits.

Carnosine is a dipeptide – beta-alanyl-L-histidine – and the beta-alanyl part comes from the non-protein-forming amino acid, beta-alanine (not alanine, as may be incorrectly stated in some commercial descriptions). Regular L-alanine is a protein-forming amino acid that we derive from the diet. The "alanine" in carnosine is different in chemical structure, does not participate in protein formation, and can interfere with membrane transport of other amino acids, especially taurine. Carnosine is similar to a slightly larger peptide, homocarnosine, and both can be synthesized in the brain in glial cells. Both are considered to have neurotransmitter functions, but homocarnosine is 100x more prevalent than carnosine in human brain. Homocarnosine, when disassembled, yields histidine and gamma-aminobutyric acid (GABA). GABA, in the brain or CNS can have calming effects and seizure-alleviating actions.

Per some clinical studies, elevated carnosine and carnosinase deficiency may or may not be coincident with neurological disorders. Carnosine levels must be balanced, and the enzyme that disassembles carnosine into histidine and beta-alanine is a zinc-dependent protein called carnosinase. Obviously, carnosinase is weak in zinc deficiency. Many autistics are reported to be low in zinc, and oral zinc supplements may or may not be effective in rectifying a functional zinc deficiency. (See section on zinc in the Minerals chapter.) My experience in looking at amino acid analyses is that carnosine is elevated in about 20% of the autistic population (before dietary and enzyme interventions). So, a carnosine-handling problem may already be in place for a subset of autistics. Oral carnosine would then be contraindicated. Probably, a 24-hour urine amino acid analysis is the most indicative test for this.

Literature – Carnosine

Chez, MG, Buchanan CP et al. "Double-blind, placebo-controlled study of L-carnosine supplementation in children with autistic spectrum disorders" *J. Child Neurol* 17 no.11 (2002) 833-837

Scriver CR and Perry TL "Disorders of α-amino acids in free and peptide-linked forms" Chapter 26 in Scriver, Beaudet et al., The Metabolic Basis of Inherited Disease 6th ed, (1989) 758-59.

Gibson KM and Jakobs C, Chapter 91 in Scriver, Beaudet et al., The Metabolic and Molecular Bases of Inherited Disease 8th ed (2001) 2097.

Item CB, Stöckler-Ipsiroglu S et al. "Arginine: glycine amidinotransferase deficiency: the third inborn error of creatine metabolism in humans" *Am J Hum Genet* 69 (2001) 1127-1133. (This is included here only because it explains the potential problem with beta-alanine.)

Creatine

Creatine is an amino acid that is involved in energy transfer, not only for muscle cells but for brain cells as well. In body tissues, creatine acts as a phosphate carrier. At the molecular level, phosphate is the currency of energy. Adding phosphate to a molecule requires an energy input, and subsequent release of phosphate releases this chemical energy. Often, the chemical reactions that occur during metabolism require an energy drive, and phosphocreatine is a long-haul transporter of needed energy. However, phosphocreatine usually doesn't interface directly with the energy-requiring reactions. Phosphorylated nucleosides like adenosine (as ATP) or guanosine (as GTP) do that. ATP and GTP are reactive, high-energy, triply-phosphated dynamos that make chemistry happen. But in many instances, the phosphate replenishment that is needed has to be delivered over distances that only phosphocreatine can traverse. The phosphocreatine energy truck uploads ADP with phosphate to make ATP, and ATP in turn uploads GDP and other nucleosides with phosphate. When we use creatine as a nutritional supplement, we're not really giving energy – we're providing a prefabricated, long distance energy carrier. For brain cells, the loaded energy carrier, phosphocreatine, provides just-in-time delivery. That's because there's very little on-hand energy stored for brain cell operation.

Indications of Need

Symptoms consistent with need include low muscle mass/strength, hypotonia, "floppy baby syndrome" in infancy, dystonic-hyperkinetic movement disorder (sometimes), seizures (sometimes), language delay, deficient expressive speech, x-linked mental retardation (sometimes), autism (sometimes). Blood creatine and urine creatinine levels have been tried as markers for creatine need and found to be problematic. Creatinine (used-up creatine in disposal form) represents less than about 3% of the total creatine inventory. Phospho-creatine is the important form, not creatine and certainly not creatinine. Unfortunately, transport of creatine can be impaired, and when this happens it gives a false impression of plentiful creatine and phosphocreatine.

Autism and mental retardation are acknowledged in medical literature to be possible outcomes of brain creatine/phosphocreatine deficiency. Creatine deficiency in the brain can result from several uncommon inborn errors of metabolism. Diagnosis of brain creatine deficit is by proton magnetic resonance spectroscopy. With autism, there is concern about creatine adequacy beyond that of uncommon inborn metabolic errors. This is because creatine formation is a SAM-methylation process (see glossary), and impaired methylation can be an acquired disorder. Elevated adenosine or adenosylhomocysteine (special lab tests) are indicators of impaired methylation and are consistent with limited levels of creatine.

When and How Much

Relatively large, therapeutic amounts of oral creatine are needed to be effective. At DAN! Conferences, clinicians reported use of amounts ranging from 300 to 1000 mg/kg body weight per day, in divided servings (doses). In a textbook-published clinical research study of individuals with a creatine synthesis deficiency, 350 to 2000 mg/kg was used (adults), and no serious side effects were found- Van Figura K, Hanefeld F et al. "Guanidoacetate Methyltransferase Deficiency" Chapter 84 in Scriver et al., Eds. The Metabolic and Molecular Bases of Inherited Disease 8th Ed. McGraw-Hill (2001) p.1903.

Because large amounts of creatine are required to gain a beneficial response, or even to do a trial to determine if there is a benefit, be sure to obtain this supplement from a reputable supplier. Small concentrations of impurities can add up when large supplemental amounts are used.

Adverse Response to Creatine?

Is it pure material? Did you get it at the local health food store where bodybuilders buy it and use it by the wheelbarrow-full? This type may not be pure enough for an autistic child whose detoxication capacity is limited.

As you read further in this chapter, you may develop considerable enthusiasm for creatine supplements. There certainly is strong circumstantial evidence of need for phosphocreatine in autism. Unfortunately, we only see notable improvement in 5 to 10% of children with ASD following creatine supplementation. We're not sure why, but we suspect problems with mitochondrial processes that make ATP which is used to load creatine with energy in the first place.

There are documented but uncommon problems in creatine transport where creatine synthesis is fine. The result can be too much creatine in the wrong place in the body. If a laboratory analysis shows high creatine, then supplementing it probably is a bad idea. One possible problem is presence of toxicants, which can stop the enzyme creatine kinase from doing its job promoting phosphocreatine formation. Phosphorylation of creatine is inhibited by mercury. Are you detoxing (mobilizing) mercury at the same time that you are using creatine? If so, phosphorylation via creatine kinase isn't going to work very well. Another acquired problem may be toxicant interference with the creatine transporter system. So, if you tried creatine early on, and it didn't work, don't discard that option permanently. It's a Tier 5 supplement because of this interference by toxicants.

About Creatine (Optional Reading)

Creatine formation in our bodies is a two step process, and I think it's important to learn a little about it because both steps are known to have inborn (genetic) problems, albeit uncommon. Additionally, creatine transport can be faulty. When any of this happens, the symptoms and impairments that result may include various autistic traits. As I described above, low creatine in the brain will result in brain cell energy deficits; one marker for this would be decreased levels of the energy dynamo, ATP – adenosine triphosphate. In 1993, Drs. Minshew, Goldstein, et al. published exactly that – low phosphocreatine and low ATP- after assessing these quantities in the frontal cortex of adolescents and young adults with autism. Nuclear magnetic resonance spectroscopy was used in a study with age, gender, race and socioeconomic status-matched controls - *Biological Psychiatry*, 1993 June <u>33</u> (11-12) pgs 762-73.

Creatine is synthesized by using parts from three amino acids, arginine (which usually is the limiting or least abundant one), glycine, and S-adenosylmethionine (SAM). In some autistics, we suspect that methylation by SAM might be restricting creatine synthesis. The first creatine synthesis step occurs primarily in the kidneys, pancreas and liver, where glycine combines with arginine to form ornithine and guanidinoacetate. The enzyme that promotes this first step of creatine synthesis is arginine-glycine amidinotransferase (AGAT). Normally, the AGAT step is the rate-limiting step of creatine synthesis, and yes, a little bit of this also happens in the brain.

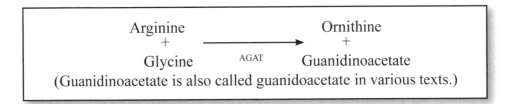

Arginine → Ornithine
+ +
Glycine AGAT Guanidinoacetate
(Guanidinoacetate is also called guanidoacetate in various texts.)

The next step is methylation by SAM using the enzyme S-adenosylmethionine-guanidinoacetate methyltransferase (GAMT). GAMT is present in brain (neurons), liver, pancreas, ovaries, testes, and epithelial tissue – so it's a very important enzyme with a very important job. In our bodies, a major part of SAM's duty is methylating guanidinoacetate to form creatine and SAH (S-adenosylhomocysteine).

SAM + Guanidinoacetate ────GAMT───→ SAH + Creatine

The SAH is where some of our biochemical worry about autism is centered. S-adenosylhomocysteine has to be metabolized into homocysteine and adenosine, and then these quantities have to be metabolized away as well. If they accumulate, as several analytical studies for autism show, then the SAH accumulates. When that happens, the GAMT enzyme can't make much creatine. Per the studies of Dr. Jill James, excessive SAH is a possibility for about one in five autistic children.

After creatine is formed, it can become an energy carrier by adding phosphate, which it acquires from ATP using the enzyme creatine kinase. Phosphocreatine then delivers high-energy phosphate some distance away where a pool of ADP needs it. This is a relatively fast and efficient way to upgrade the distant ADP to ATP. Besides the two enzymatic steps of creatine formation, AGAT and GAMT, another molecular process is crucial to the supply of creatine and phosphate. That process is accomplished by the "creatine transporter" (CRTR, or CRT in some texts). Intercellular transport of creatine is needed to get it from places of assembly to places of usage. At this writing, the exact configuration of the creatine transporter system has not been described. It is suspected to be similar to the transporters that work for GABA, serotonin, dopamine, and taurine.

Under normal physiologic conditions, about 1% of creatine and about 2-3% of phosphocreatine are lost to creatinine per day. Creatinine is a final waste product of energy and amino acid metabolism, and it's excreted in urine. That's why continual, daily makeup of some new creatine is required.

Creatinine is often used by laboratories as a yardstick against which "spot" urine samples are ratioed. Unfortunately, many autistic children have been found to have low creatinine. Mathematically, when you ratio a normal result to low creatinine, you get the appearance of a "high" result. This means that you can get some very misleading answers from that lab test. DO NOT believe these answers unless the measured creatinine level is normal considering age and sex. If the patient is a child, be sure the lab used a child's reference range. This is one reason why a 24-hour urine test is vastly more reliable and indicative than a "spot" test.

Very significant amounts of creatine and phosphocreatine are normally found in brain. Much of the brain's energy consumption is for cellular communication processes. This includes signal transduction between neurons (synaptic processes), signal transduction across the neuronal membranes and the attendant processes of chemical change within brain cells. Energy is transferred, changed in form and consumed by perceiving, thinking and responding. There's more about this in the Guanosine section of the Glossary.

Once again, documented metabolic errors are associated with all three creatine formation and delivery processes, AGAT, GAMT, and the CRTR gene. And all three defects produce delayed development of speech, lack of expressive speech, and sometimes other autistic traits. Often, there are seizures as well.

Literature - Creatine

Minshew NJ, Goldstein G, Dobrowski SM, et al. "A preliminary 31P MRS study of autism: evidence for undersynthesis and increased degradation of brain membranes. *Biol Psychiatry* 1993 June 1-5, 33(11-12):762-73

Von Figura K, Hanefeld F et al. "Guanidinoacetate Methyltransferase Deficiency" Chapter 84 in Scriver et al., eds., The Metabolic and Molecular Gases of Inherited Disease 8th Ed., McGraw-Hill (2001) 1903.

Wyss M and Kaddurah-Daouk R "Creatine and Creatinine Metabolism" *Physiological Reviews* 80 no.3 (2000) 1113-1114.

Martin DW "Contractile & Structural Proteins" Chapt. 34 in Martin DW, Mayes PA et al. eds., Harper's Review of Biochemistry 20th ed, Lange Medical Publications (1985) 488.

Granner DK "Hormone Action" Chapter 44 in Murray RK, Granner DK et al. Harper's Biochemistry 25th ed., (2000) 541-544.

Salomons GS, van Dooren SJM et al. "X-linked creatine transporter (SLC6A8) defect: a new creatine deficiency syndrome" *Am.J.Human Genetics* 68 (2001) 1497-1500.

Salomons GS, van Dooren SJM et al. "X-linked creatine transporter defect: an overview" *J. Inherited Metabolic Disorders* 26 (2003) 309-318.

Item CB, Stöckler-Ipsiroglu S et al. "Arginine: Glycine Amidinotransferase Deficiency: The third inborn error of creatine metabolism in humans" *Am.J.Human Genetics* 69 (2001) 1127-1133.

Digestive Enzymes

Digestive enzyme supplements contain plant or animal source proteins that are analogs of human enzymes, meaning that they have similar or identical digestive properties for the foods that we eat. My efforts on enzyme formulation dates from about 1990, when I noticed the frequent presence of small peptides (anserine, carnosine) in the urine of some autistics. Working with Gary Osborn of Apothecure Pharmacy, Dallas, we came up with a peptidase that seemed to help. At the first DAN! Conference (January 1995), Dr. Karl Reichelt of Norway provided much more incentive for enzyme use. He presented clinical laboratory findings about opiate-acting peptides of grain and dairy food sources in autistics' urine. These peptides are a bit bigger, five to nine amino acids long, and they have undesired biologic activity that goes beyond the possibility of opiate action. Further findings (1999-2005) by Drs. Horvath et al., Kushak, Buie, and Winter, point to problems in carbohydrate digestion for many with ASD. This has led to a selection of digestive enzyme products from several manufacturers tailored especially for the needs of individuals with ASD. The March 2009 ARI Parent Response Tally for Digestive Enzymes (n=2350) is: benefit for 62%, no effect for 35%, worsening for 3%. In my opinion, diet adjustment and digestive enzyme supplementation are the best ways to start nutritional intervention for at least 60% of children and adults with ASD. This is Tier 1 activity.

Indications of Need

All of the following are consistent with need for digestive supplements with meals: food sensitivities or reactivities, detoxification therapies, bowel irregularity, abnormal stools, gastrointestinal distress or behaviors consistent with abdominal discomfort, irritable bowel syndrome, colitis (inflammation in the colon), elevated inflammatory markers related to intestinal disorder (cytokines such as TNFα), intestinal dysbiosis, and signs of maldigestion including increased stool fat content per stool analysis.

When, How Much, and Which Ones?

Let's tackle the last question first – which enzymes? Except for stool fat content (short-chain or long-chain fatty acids or cholesterol) measured by stool analysis, practical, clinical lab tests to determine need for specific digestive enzymes remain an unmet necessity. At present, there is a laboratory in Norway developing a test for the opiate-like peptides (casomorphins, gluteomorphins); a urine specimen is required. Assessment of carbohydrate digestive enzyme insufficiency is a clinical investigation that requires biopsy of the mucosal tissue of the small intestine.

I think the best bet is a comprehensive enzyme supplement that includes proteases (digest proteins), peptidases (digest the peptide pieces of proteins), carbohydrate digesters including amylases and disaccharidases, and lipase for dietary fat.

When? Digestive enzymes formulated for those with ASD are almost all designed to be taken at the beginning of each meal. These enzymes start their work in the stomach and continue working as partially-digested food passes into the small intestine. Most of their work is done and they are themselves broken down before exiting the small intestine. There is no evidence that supplemental enzymes are absorbed intact into the bloodstream. They are proteins from plants or animals and are themselves digested like food. Skipping digestive enzymes at a meal can be bad news, because partially-digested food can feed unfriendly flora and lead to dysbiosis, inflammation and toxicant uptake. This can have long-term effects.

How much?

This depends upon how much food is eaten, not how big the person is. Here, you should follow the manufacturer's instructions on the label or the instructions from your doctor or nutrition counselor. There is little uniformity in potency per serving for enzymes across brands, and the specific types (and sources) of enzyme materials can vary as well.

Adverse Response to Digestive Enzymes?

The general rule is to follow the manufacturer's or provider's instructions for use. Most of the enzymes offered for autism are plant-based. Some come from highly refined aspergillus strains, and the refining has removed the allergenic substances that used to be a problem with supplements from this source. Nevertheless, do a trial with just one capsule before a meal to check for tolerance. Use of digestive enzymes can provoke temporary symptoms which I will discuss below. These symptoms usually appear after a day or two of enzyme use and may continue for a week to two weeks. So tolerance or intolerance to enzymes can be difficult to judge initially. Expect to have a period of "worse before better".

When digestive enzymes with DPP4 are used, the exposure to dietary opiate peptides is decreased as casein and gluten peptides are digested by the enzymes. This usually brings about a period of opiate-like withdrawal, which may last 5 to 10 days or longer in some cases. During this period, the individual may become irritable or tantrum, develop hyperactivity, experience an increase in stimming, or present increased levels of inappropriate behavior or regression. Cravings for discontinued foods often occur. Not all children experience withdrawal or adverse reactions when starting the enzymes. Prior elimination of casein foods from the diet significantly lessens or might eliminate withdrawal symptoms that occur initially with enzyme use, but then you'll get similar symptoms at the beginning of the casein-free diet. Experience tells us to start the enzymes gradually, and do it before starting diet trials.

Decreasing undigested food in the lower gastrointestinal tract can lower or eliminate a food supply that might have fostered the growth of dysbiotic, possibly pathogenic flora. Autistics often have increased permeability of the gut wall, which allows an increased toxic burden. A temporary result of digestive enzyme use can be die-off of dysbiotic flora with consequent release of even more toxins. The die-off period usually does not last more than a week, but may continue longer with persistent, adaptable dysbiotic strains. You'll get after these strains during Tier 2.

If the period of adverse response to digestive enzymes continues beyond two weeks, please consult your doctor or health professional. There's no harm in stopping the enzyme supplement to investigate what's going wrong. Clinical laboratory tests can be informative in cases of prolonged problems – a comprehensive diagnostic stool analysis, an amino acid analysis (24-hour urine collection is preferred for this situation), and a food allergy workup. Food allergies can cause inflammation of the intestinal mucosa and worsening of the responses described above. Better digestion typically reduces but does not necessarily eliminate food allergy symptoms.

Also, a capsule of activated charcoal, taken three times per day (away from meds and supplements) may reduce or stop "die-off" symptoms. Charcoal does this by absorbing toxins from dysbiotic flora before the toxins can cross into the bloodstream. It does not, however, significantly reduce withdrawal symptoms.

About Digestive Enzymes (Optional Reading)

While the diet is being adjusted or just before, you should give digestive enzymes a try, understanding at the outset that digestive enzymes are not a substitute for a special or exclusionary diet. Make only one change at a time.

Will enzymes obscure the effects of the CF, GF and SCD trials? To some degree they will. For autistics, the three primary purposes of supplemented enzymes are: (1) to break apart or digest peptides that could be absorbed and lead to disruption of cellular perception and response processes, (2) to reduce or shut off inappropriate food supply to the lower small intestine and large bowel, i.e. the food supply for dysbiotic flora, and (3) to reduce food allergy symptoms. Supplemental enzymes cannot be depended upon to be 100% effective in finding and digesting all of the peptide and disaccharide molecules. Even with digestive enzyme use, you'll usually be able to see further benefits of excluding dietary casein or gluten foods.

Digestive enzymes, the natural ones in our gastrointestinal tracts and the supplemental ones that come in capsules, are proteins that have the catalytic ability to disassemble large food molecules. Digestive enzyme supplements come from plant or animal sources (classified legally as "foods"), and they can help us to digest food when they are taken with a meal. The different types of digestive enzymes include: proteases for breaking proteins down into peptides, and peptidases for breaking peptides down to individual, free-form amino acids or short-chain peptides. Short-chain peptides are dipeptides (two amino acids linked together) and perhaps some tripeptides (three amino acids linked together). Lipases split dietary fat molecules into smaller pieces (glycerol and fatty acids). Amylases break dietary starch down into simpler carbohydrates like disaccharides or monosaccharide sugars. Sometimes additional enzymes are present that break down the cellular structure of plants – cellulases, hemicellulase and xylanases. Disaccharidases break complex sugars down into simple sugars. We often need disaccharidase help in autism: lactase (for processing milk sugar into glucose and galactose), and maltase and isomaltase for processing some complex sugars into simple ones like glucose or fructose. When nutritional supplements are needed, digestive enzyme supplements are usually needed also, because they improve the body's ability to extract nutrients from food.

Dipeptidylpeptidase-IV

A natural peptidase enzyme of particular interest in autism is dipeptidylpeptidase IV (DPP4). DPP4's job is to break apart peptides that have the amino acid proline at every other position in the peptide molecule. Such peptides, "exorphins," have morphine-like action on neuronal cells. Beta-casomorphin 7 from casein is such a peptide:

Tyrosine-proline-phenylalanine-proline-glycine-proline-isoleucine

DPP4 cleaves peptides such as these at the second bond (a proline-amino acid bond) from the nitrogen-terminal end (the left end as written). Thus, DPP4 acting successively on beta-casomorphin 7 causes:

Tyr-Pro / Phe-Pro-Gly-Pro-Ile
Tyr-Pro / Phe-Pro / Gly-Pro-Ile
Tyr-Pro / Phe-Pro / Gly-Pro / Ile

In the human digestive tract, only DPP4 can do this. But like many enzymes, DPP4 is subject to inactivation or poisoning by external substances. During the 1980s and 1990s, Drs. Reichelt, Cade and others found undigested exorphin peptides in the urine of autistics. These findings are consistent with impaired and deficient activity of DPP4. In 1982, Püschel et al. examined human placental DPP4 and found that it is inactivated by mercury, organophosphates (pesticide sprays), zinc and cadmium chlorides, and lead acetate.

Here, we've come upon another reason for supplementing digestive enzymes – to compensate for certain toxic exposures or contaminations. Such exposures may be an underlying cause of some of the traits found in autistics. During detoxification therapy, circulating toxicants can increase the need for enzyme supplements.

Why do we need to get rid of these casomorphin peptides? An obvious reason is their opiate activity, when absorbed into the bloodstream via a too-permeable intestinal lining. A less obvious reason is that they might interfere with the workings of the DPP4 protein elsewhere in the body. On the surface of some immune cells, this same protein is a signaling agent, cluster differentiation factor 26 (CD26). Casomorphins bind to DPP4 and they could bind to CD26, too: see Vojdani et al., *Int J Immunopath and Pharmacol* 16 no.3 (2003) 189-199. Some cell membranes contain DPP4 as a protein which anchors an enzyme that processes adenosine (see Glossary). Per the clinical research of Dr. Jill James, about 20% of autistic children feature elevated adenosine (not good). One consequence is impaired methylation (also not good). Can casomorphins bind to DPP4 and disrupt its job as an anchor for the adenosine deaminase enzyme? I don't know, but why else is adenosine high in one out of five untreated autistics?

My advice is to use digestive enzyme products that include plant analog DPP4 to knock out the casomorphin peptides and eliminate the potential opiate and adenosine problems.

Aids for Carbohydrate Digestion

Now, let's switch to carbohydrate digestion, which has been found faulty in autistics by several gastroenterologists and researchers in enzymology. Lactase, which digests the milk sugar lactose, is the disaccharidase enzyme that is most often weak in autistics. Lactose, a disaccharide sugar, is glucose attached to galactose. It's these simple sugars (glucose, fructose, galactose) that are absorbed; with normal gut permeability, disaccharides and complex sugars are not absorbed. Lactase in the small intestine separates lactose into glucose and galactose. Lactase is most active in mildly acidic conditions (pH or 5.5 to 6.0). To make this work, the pancreas has to put adequate bicarbonate into the much more acidic food matter coming from the stomach. For whatever reason, though, lactase deficiency is present in at least 60% of tested autistics. So, lactase must also be in digestive enzyme formulations for use in autism.

Three other disaccharide sugars also are known to be not digested well by autistics:

> Maltose: glucose + glucose with a $1 \to 4$ glycosidic bond
> Isomaltose: glucose + glucose with a $1 \to 6$ glycosidic bond-
> Palatinose: glucose + fructose with a $1 \to 6$ glycosidic bond

The difference between maltose and isomaltose is how their two component sugars are linked together. Two different digestive enzymes, maltase and isomaltase, are needed, one for each. Palatinose uses the isomaltase enzyme for digestion. Because many autistics have maltase and isomaltase/palatinase deficiencies too, these also need to be provided as supplemental digestive enzymes.

Finally, a few words about lipase, the digestive enzyme that breaks complicated dietary fats into two types of molecules that can be absorbed more easily – fatty acids and glycerol. For years, we saw elevated fats in the stools of autistics when a stool or digestive stool analysis was done. At the Atlanta DAN! Conference in May 2001, Jeff Bradstreet M.D. (Melbourne, FL) spoke about this. Over 50% of his autistic patients showed some degree of excessive stool fat per the Great Smokies Diagnostic Lab (now Genova Diagnostics) CDSA test. Other labs now also offer this test. When this problem gets bad enough (steatorrhea), fatty acid, vitamin D and calcium deficiencies can occur. Then oxalate excess can also be a problem see Calcium section of the Minerals chapter. The temporary, and sometimes long-term, remedy is to provide lipase orally with meals.

Literature – Digestive Enzymes

Reichelt KL, Ekrem J and Scott H "Gluten, Milk Proteins and Autism: Dietary Intervention Effects on Behavior and Peptide Secretion" *J.Appl. Nutrition* 42 no.1 (1990). 1-11.

Reichelt KL, Knivsberg AM et al. "Nature and Consequences of Hyperpeptiduria and Bovine Casomorphins Found in Autistic Syndromes" *Dev. Brain Dysfunct* 7 (1994) 71-85.

Cade R, Privette M et al. "Autism and Schizophrenia: Intestinal Disorders" *Nutritional Neuroscience* 3 (2000) 57-72.

Püschel G, Mentlein R and Heymann E "Isolation and Characterization of Dipeptidyl Peptidase IV from Human Placenta" *Eur. J. Biochem* 126 (1982) 359-365.

Vojdani A, Pangborn JB et al. "Infections, toxic chemicals and dietary peptides binding to lymphocyte receptors and tissue enzymes are major instigators of autoimmunity in autism" *Int.J.Immunopath and Pharmacol* 16 no.3 (2003) 189-199.

Horvath K, Papdimitriou JC et al. "Gastrointestinal abnormalities in children with autistic disorder" *J. Pediatrics* 135 no.5 (1999) 559-563.

Horvath K and Perman JA "Autistic disorder and gastrointestinal disease" *Curr. Opinion in Pediatrics* 14 (2002) 583-387.

Kushak RI and Buie T "Disaccharidase deficiencies in patients with autistic spectrum disorders" presented at the DAN! New Orleans Think Tank, January 2004.

Brudnak MA, Rimland B et al. "Enzyme-based therapy for autism spectrum disorders – is it worth another look?" *Medical Hypotheses* (2002 58 5) 422-426

Kushak RI, Winter HAS et al. "Gastrointestinal symptoms and intestinal disaccharidase activities in children with autism" N.Am.Soc. Pediatric Gastroenterology, Hepatology and Nutrition, Oct 2005, Salt Lake City, Poster paper. Dr. Rafael Kushak, Mass General Hospital for Children, Harvard Medical School, Boston MA, Pediatric GI Unit.

Dimethylglycine, Trimethylglycine (Betaine)

Just as the names indicate, dimethylglycine (DMG) is the amino acid glycine with two attached methyls, and the tri- (TMG) has three methyls. What's a methyl? Please refer to the Glossary. Metabolically and nutritionally, the tri-form comes from choline (which is now classified as nutritionally essential), and the di- form results after the tri-form gives away one of its methyls. What we hope is that it went to homocysteine to (re) make methionine. Trimethylglycine is the same as 'betaine", which also is called "glycine betaine". Dimethylglycine and trimethylglycine are of physiologic value to those with ASD who can derive benefit from increased methylation of homocysteine to form (more) methionine. Just as supplementing methionine or S-adenosylmethionine is chancy and not recommended early on, I don't recommend use of either DMG or TMG until you arrive at Tier 4 or preferably Tier 5 of the Intervention Schedule.

Indications of Need

Behaviorally and functionally, it's hard to separate DMG and TMG in terms of need. When one or the other works, reports from parents overwhelmingly point to improved verbal communication. There is also clear evidence that DMG is the one to start with, because the adverse responses to TMG (16%, n=1132) are twice that of DMG (8%, n=6363). Some of the adverse responses, in my opinion, are due to trying them too early in the intervention program.

Some nutritional supplement manufacturers provide DMG and TMG with added folate (or folinic acid) and vitamin B_{12}. That's because folate and B_{12} are needed when DMG is disassembled metabolically in the body to provide chemical parts that go into the assembly of methylated tetrahydrofolate (THF). Methylated THF and vitamin B_{12} work together to methylate homocysteine and make methionine. A behavioral indication of need for B_{12} and folate with either TMG or DMG is hyperactivity.

Analytical indications that DMG with folate and B_{12} might be beneficial –

- An amino acid analysis with low cystine, cysteine or cyst(e)ine and with low or low-normal methionine
- Adenosylhomocysteine and homocysteine are not elevated.
- A vitamin analysis indicating low folate
- Metabolic analyses showing high "FIGlu" or high "MMA"
- A hair element analysis showing deficient cobalt (Cobalt is the element that activates vitamin B_{12}, cobalamin.)

Analytical indications that TMG with folate and vitamin B_{12} might be beneficial –

- An amino acid analysis with elevated adenosylhomocysteine, homocysteine, homocysteine, or homocyst(e)ine
- An amino acid analysis showing methionine and/or SAM deficiency
- Metabolic analysis or organic acid analysis showing high urine "FIGlu" or high urine "MMA"
- A vitamin analysis indicating low folate
- A hair element analysis showing deficient cobalt (cobalt activates B_{12}, cobalamin)

Sometimes, clinicians or nutritionists attempt to use laboratory test results and behaviors to judge whether DMG or TMG would be the better supplement. My procedure for judging this is to score a dozen or so factors as shown below.

DMG-TMG Choice Matrix

	DMG	DMG + Fol.+B_{12}*	TMG	TMG+ Fol. + B_{12}
Poor speech development	x	x	x	x
Poor eye contact	x	x	x	x
Has hyperactivity		x		x
Cystine or cysteine is low	x		x	
Homocystine is high				x
Methionine and/or SAM is low			x	x
Histidine is high	x			
Folate is high	x		x	
Reacts to folate	x		x	
Folate is low		x		x
Urine "FIGlu" high**		x		x
B_{12} shots worsen	x		x	
Low cobalt per hair element analysis		x		x
Urine "MMA" high		x		x

Add up all the x's that apply. Whichever product gets the most x's is your first choice. If you get fewer than two x's for each of the four possible products, then it is not likely that any of the four will be of great benefit. If you get a tie between DMG and DMG + Folate+ B_{12}, make DMG your first choice. If you get a tie between TMG and TMG + Folate + B_{12}, choose TMG. If you get a tie between DMG and TMG, choose DMG. However, no formula is infallible. The right product is the one that the individual does the best with.

*The new generation of these supplements uses folinic acid and methylcobalamin

**Impairments in purine synthesis or unusual folate traps may cause FIGlu to be elevated regardless of supplemental forms of folate/B_{12}.

When and How Much?

If you're at Tier 5 and speech hasn't happened yet, or if it's only echolalia, then this is the time to try DMG, then maybe TMG.

The suggested continual supplement range for DMG is tabulated below, and even higher amounts may be beneficial and may be recommended by your physician. At one of the DAN! Conferences, one parent reported great success with 2000 mg/d (16 tablets over a 24-hour period) for a 15-year old autistic. Do not try such high amounts on your own – have your doctor involved.

Body Weight	DMG Daily Servings *
Lb/Kg	Range, mg/d
44/20	125-375
66/30	190-560
88/40	250-750
110/50	300-900
132/60	375-1100
154/70	450-1300

*This is approximately the range that corresponds to the Parent Tally statistics, below. More may be given if medically advised.

Dimethylglycine Parent Response Rally, Responses, n =6363, ARI Publ.34/March 2009		
Behavior or Traits Improved	No Discernible Effect	Behavior or Traits Worsened
42%	50%	8%

The suggested continual supplement range for TMG is tabulated below, and here again, higher amounts have been used by some parents/doctors with reported success.

Body Weight	TMG Daily Servings *
Lb/Kg	Range, mg/d
44/20	150-500
66/30	250-800
88/40	350-1050
110/50	450-1300
132/60	550-1600
154/70	600-2000

*This is approximately the range that corresponds to Parent Tally statistics shown below.

Recent clinical research by Dr. Jill James shows that after TMG (and folinic acid) supplementation, the ratio of reduced to oxidized glutathione improves – less of the oxidized and more of the active reduced form. This indicates that TMG is helping to relieve the methionine-methylation hangup as it increases levels of methionine, SAM and glutathione.

Trimethylglycine Parent Response Rally, Responses, n =6363, ARI Publ.34/March 2009		
Behavior or Traits Improved	No Discernible Effect	Behavior or Traits Worsened
41%	43%	16%

Adverse Response to DMG?

As tabulated above, eight out of 100 individuals on the autistic spectrum have "trouble" with DMG. Usually this trouble is more stimming or hyperactivity. Biochemically, there are two circumstances that we know of that could cause problems. The first is that folate, as tetrahydrofolate, is insufficient or unable to accept and utilize the one-carbon chemical pieces that DMG provides. Supplementing folinic acid and vitamin B_{12} as methylcobalamin along with DMG may solve the problem. If none of the DMG formulations help, then discontinue it and try TMG.

Adverse Response to TMG?

Are you also using taurine? If not, start the trial over after taurine has been used for a week or so, and continue the taurine while TMG is used. Are you using betaine•HCl? Don't, it's too acidic. The name and synonyms of what you should be using are: trimethylglycine, betaine, glycine-betaine, oxyneurine, and lycine. What you should not be using is betaine hydrochloride, betaine HCl, pluchine or trimethylglycine hydrochloride.

Because TMG becomes DMG and DMG needs tetrahydrofolate directly and vitamin B_{12} indirectly, TMG may not be beneficial without supplementing folate (or folinic acid) and vitamin B_{12} as well.

About TMG and DMG (Optional Reading)

Tri- and dimethylglycine are natural biochemicals in our bodies, forming a chemical link between cholinergic processes and methionine metabolism (methylation and transsulfuration). Put more simply, material that's left over from important neurotransmitter and nervous system work becomes a source of chemical parts that are needed for antioxidant work, detoxication, genetic expression, immune response and neuronal synchrony. So, DMG and TMG are pretty important and some with ASD just don't have enough of them.

TMG comes from choline. When choline is made in the body it requires lots of chemical energy and lots of SAM-methylation. Normally, we don't make enough ourselves, so food-source choline was finally declared to be an essential nutrient in 1998 by the Food & Nutrition Board, Institute of Medicine. With the reduced SAM methylation that we've discovered in a subset of ASD individuals, choline becomes even more important. But even more useful to us is trimethylglycine (betaine), which comes from choline. It's trimethyl glycine, TMG, that methylates homocysteine to form methionine – a methylation route that duplicates what methyl-tetrahydrofolate, vitamin B_{12} (cobalamin) and methionine synthase also do.

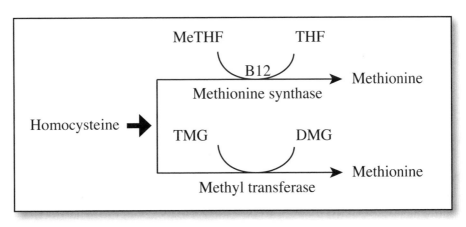

There is a problem that can arise if we get too enthusiastic about changing our homocysteine back into methionine. The problem is that only about a third or perhaps half of our homocysteine is supposed to be recycled to methionine. The rest has to go to make cysteine, glutathione, sulfate, taurine, etc. We might get along for awhile with limited cysteine, GSH and sulfate (many with ASD are limited in these), but limited taurine gets serious because it can lead to seizures. This may already be going on in some with ASD, and you don't want to make it worse by overdoing TMG supplements. So, have the taurine supplement ongoing when you try TMG. But before you try TMG, or TMG with B_{12} and folinic acid, or whatever, try DMG first.

Dimethylglycine used to be part of a concoction called "pangamic acid" or vitamin B_{15}. The "vitamin" classification was (and is) erroneous, and neither pangamic acid nor B_{15} was a pure substance.

DMG doesn't let go of its methyl parts as easily as TMG does. Instead, DMG is disassembled to form a one-carbon part (formic acid) plus an amino acid called sarcosine. Sarcosine then comes apart to make glycine plus more formic acid. Formic acid gets transformed to methylene, and that's added to THF (tetrahydrofolate). Eventually, this becomes methyl THF. That methyl part is what goes to cobalamin on methionine synthase; see the diagram above. The DMG process is more involved, more controlled and probably more gradual in methylating homocysteine than is the TMG process.

The formic acid pieces from DMG also go in another metabolic direction. Formyl THF and methylene THF are used in the synthesis of "purines", the basic molecules that become adenosine and AMP, ADP, ATP (adenosine mono, di, tri phosphate) and also guanosine, and GMP, GDP, GTP, etc. These molecules are fundamental to health and life – more reason for the importance of choline, TMG and DMG.

Literature – DMG and TMG (Betaine)

Graber CD et al. "Immunomodulating Properties of Dimethylglycine in Humans" *J.Infect.Dis* (143(1), (Jan 1981) 101-105

Kern JK et al. "Effectiveness of N,N-dimethylglycine in autism and pervasive developmental disorder" *J.Child Neurol* 16(3) Mar 2001, 169-73

James SJ et al. "Metabolic biomarkers of increased oxidative stress and impaired methylation capacity in children with autism" *Am J Clin Nutr* 80(6) Dec 2004, 1611-17

Fatty Acids

The cells in our bodies have protective membranes that enclose them, "cell walls", as they're sometimes called. A cell's wall is really a membrane composed of fatty acids which keeps water-soluble stuff, toxins and microorganisms outside and separated from the special water-soluble substances inside. The inside of a cell has many compartments and centers of activity such as the mitochondria, Golgi complexes and lysosomes; these are also separated and contained by lipid membranes. The cell wall/membrane is a double layer of fatty acids, as are mitochondrial walls. Lysosomes and Golgi complexes have single-thickness fatty acid membranes which are not completely continuous. They have channels for nutrients and wastes to pass in and out, and they have binding sites (proteins) where messengers can dock in order to signal the cell about external happenings and requirements. Our body builds these membranes out of fatty acids that it processes from dietary sources. In autism, cell membrane composition is especially important because the kinds of fatty acids adjacent to messenger binding sites have a strong effect on message transmission and cellular understanding of external events.

Most infants and children with ASD benefit from supplemental essential fatty acids of the "omega-3" type (see following, About Fatty Acids). Laboratory analysis of red blood cell (erythrocyte) fatty acids is available if you'd like analytical confirmation of need. Such tests are not always indicative, because they don't assess the membrane makeup of other cell types, such as neurons, where problems may be occurring.

Indications of Need

Overt symptoms that are consistent with need for fatty acids supplements include: dry, chapped or scaly skin or lips, atopic eczema, areas of tiny bumps on the back of upper arms, dry or itchy eyes, frequent thirst, finger/toe nails that chip or fray easily, and frequent infections (this and skin bumpiness may also be due to insufficient vitamin A).

When and How Much?

While we do not have parent response tallies for improvement vs. worsening with fatty acid supplements, we do have many testimonial reports of benefits from their use with autistics. Levels of both omega-3 (especially) and omega-6 types can be depressed in this population, as measured by erythrocyte membrane analyses. Perhaps this is consistent with elevated fats in stools of autistics who are not taking lipase enzymes. A common abnormality in autism is a depressed level of omega-3 fatty acids, especially docosahexaenoic acid, DHA. I suggest you start early on with a supplement of unsaturated fatty acids containing omega-3 types. The end of Tier 1 should be okay for such a supplement.

There are some sensible prerequisites to the use of fatty acid supplements. Usually, a supplement of taurine is beneficial and occasionally glycine as well. These amino acids are needed to make bile salts, which emulsify and make conjugates and "micelles" of dietary fats and fatty acids. This process is necessary for uptake of most lipid nutrients from the small intestine. Without adequate amounts of bile salts, fatty acid supplements can, like fats in food, pass right on through without being absorbed.

Amounts of omega-3 fatty acids that have been helpful range from 20 to 40 mg per Kg of body weight. So, a 24 Kg (55 lb) child would be expected to benefit from 400 to 1000 mg/day of omega-3 fatty acids., Often, the omega-3 portion of a fatty acid capsule is only 25 to 35%, so it may take three or four 1000-mg soft-gel capsules to provide 1000 mg of omega-3 fatty acids. DHA is only a fraction of the omega-3 content, 30 to 50% in most supplement products. Thus, three 1000-mg soft-gel omega-3 fatty acid capsules usually provide about 300-500 mg of DHA, which usually is adequate.

Adverse Responses to Fatty Acids?

Problems with fatty acid supplements are uncommon, and are usually related to spoilage. Puncture or break open a capsule and smell it. It should smell fresh. If it smells rancid, toss out the lot, or return it and request a refund. Also, always check and respect the expiration date or "best if used before" date on fatty acid/essential oil packaging. Beware of products without such dates. Keep fatty acid supplement bottles refrigerated before and after opening.

Giving too much at one time can cause intestinal or bowel symptoms including gas for some people. Start with one capsule/day and work up to the desired amount. Also, ensure by product label or contact with the supplier that fish oil fatty acids are "mercury free" (less than detectable by analysis).

About Fatty Acids (Optional Reading)

Fatty acids come in many varieties, some from the diet and many made or altered in body tissues. These molecules are chains of carbon atoms with an organic acid group, a carboxyl group, -COOH at one end, and a methyl group, -CH$_3$ on the other end. Chemists number these carbon atoms, starting with the carbon in the carboxyl group as number "one". The last carbon at the opposite end of the chain, the one in the methyl group, either has a number or is referred to generically as the "omega" (ω) carbon. The names of fatty acids typically refer to the total number of included carbon atoms. For example, decanoic acid (10 carbons) is:

$$CH3CH2CH2CH2CH2CH2CH2CH2CH2COOH.$$

Because of its electron structure, each carbon atom has four arms or bonds that it uses to attach to other atoms. Methane, for example, is CH$_4$, a carbon atom holding on to four hydrogen atoms. In the fatty acid chain shown above, except for the ends, each carbon holds another carbon on each side plus two hydrogens. This structure is called "saturated"; the carbons are holding onto all that they possibly can. It results in straight-chain molecules that stack together easily, forming solid shapes rather than flexible membranes. At body temperature, saturated fatty acids with chains containing more than 10 carbons are solids if they are grouped together (decanoic acid melts at 30°C, dodecanoic or lauric acid with 12 carbons melts at 44°C, while octanoic acid with eight carbons melts at 16°C and is a liquid at usual room temperatures).

Cells can't live with solid, inflexible sheets of fat for a membrane. Instead, they are composed mostly of flexible, "unsaturated" fatty acids. In unsaturated fatty acids, two or four or six or more of the carbons are joined in pairs by double bonds. These kinds of fatty acids are called "polyunsaturated" fatty acids or "PUFA"s. In order to have this, some hydrogen atoms are omitted. An important fatty acid in cell membranes, docosahexaenoic acid or DHA, has 22 carbons with six pairs of double-bonded carbons. In the shorthand nomenclature of chemists, DHA is 22:6ω3, and the first of the six double bonds starts at the third carbon from the omega end. (Sorry, I didn't make up this nomenclature; it's traditional chemistry.) Here's a simple diagram of DHA's carbon (C), hydrogen (H) and oxygen (O) structure.

22 21 20 19 18 17 16 15 14 13 12 11 10 9 8 7 6 5 4 3 2 1
CH3CH2CH=CHCH2CH=CHCH2CH=CHCH2CH=CHCH2CH=CHCH2CH=CHCH2CH2COOH

DHA is a very important and abundant lipid in brain tissue. In cell membranes, it contributes to fluidity, correct receptor function and interaction with lipid hormones such as estrogen, progesterone, and angiotensin. Cell membrane fatty acids are those with 18 to as many as 24 carbons, and most of them are unsaturated to some extent.

Unsaturated fatty acids have flexibility, and they actually have angles or kinks in their shape. (This isn't shown in the straight-line simplification above.) The two major types of membrane fatty acids are the omega-3 types (which DHA is), and the omega-6 type. Some omega-3s are:

Alpha-linolenic	18:3Ω3
Eicosapentaenoic	20:5Ω3
Docosapentaenoic	22:5Ω3
Docosahexaenoic	22:6Ω3

Some omega-6s are:

Linoleic	18:2Ω6
Gamma-linolenic	18:3Ω6
Dihomo-Gamma-linolenic	20:3Ω6
Arachidonic	20:4Ω6

Literature - Fatty Acids

Pastural E et al. "Novel plasma phospholipid biomarkers of autism: mitochondrial dysfunction as a putative causative mechanism" *Prostaglandins Leukot Essent Fatty Acids*, 2009 Jul 14.

Kitajka K et al. "Effects of dietary omega-3 polyunsaturated fatty acids on brain gene expression" *PNAS* 0402342101 July 27, 2004 vol 101 no. 30 10931-36

Horrobin DF Clinical Uses of Essential Fatty Acids Eden Press 1982. Out of print, but excellent and may be available from libraries.

Bazan N, Murphy M and Toffano G Neurobiology of Essential Fatty Acids Plenum Press, 1992 – Advances in Experimental Medicine and Biology Series vol. 318 (technical, for doctors/researchers)

Sinn N, Bryan J, Wilson C "Cognitive effects of polyunsaturated fatty acids in children with attention deficit hyperactivity disorder symptoms: A randomized controlled trial" *Prostaglandins, Leukotrienes and Essential Fatty Acids* 78 (2008) 311-326.

Glutathione

In the last two and a half decades, the natural tripeptide, glutathione, has become one of the most popular topics for clinical and nutritional study with over 60,000 citations listed on the Internet in "Pub Med" alone. Glutathione influences detoxication, oxidant/antioxidant balance, immune response, insulin, glucose metabolism, transport of nutrients across membranes, and mediation of inflammation. It is required for metabolism of vitamin B_{12}. Frequently glutathione has been measured to be subnormal in blood or erythrocytes of autistics and too much of it is in the inactive, oxidized form.

Indications of Need

Cellular (erythrocyte) levels of active glutathione (GSH) and oxidized (inactive) glutathione (GSSG) can be measured by clinical laboratories. Any decrease in GSH or increase in GSSG beyond laboratory norms is an indication of need for GSH. Lower-than-normal levels of other antioxidants such as vitamin C or vitamin E can indicate need for supplemental GSH. Abnormal amino acid results can be consistent with need: methionine excess/deficiency, homocysteine excess, cystine/cysteine deficiency in plasma, cystinuria (high urine cystine) and other aminoacidopathies of transsulfuration/transmethylation. (These are medical issues requiring consultation with health professionals). Magnesium deficiency is consistent with need for supplemental GSH because it is needed by the enzymes that assemble it.

Also consistent with need are: chronic or episodic signs of oxidant stress/inflammation, known exposure to environmental toxicant chemicals, past exposure to toxic elements, especially mercury. In my opinion, autism spectrum disorder is a condition that warrants trial use of glutathione, but not until Tier 4 of the nutritional intervention schedule.

When and How Much?

The *when* for oral GSH supplements is after the intestinal tract is cleaned up and contains a populace of normal and friendly flora, and when you (and your doctor) decide it's time to emphasize detoxication or do detoxification treatments. You will almost certainly get in trouble by using oral glutathione while dysbiotic flora still reign in the gut. (An optional medical procedure to get around this is intravenous infusion of GSH – consult your doctor.)

How much depends upon how well the body is doing at making NADPH, the hydrogen source for recycling oxidized glutathione, GSSG, to regenerate GSH. It also depends on the amount and type of sequestered toxicants in body tissues, especially mercury and arsenic, and how much of the other antioxidant team members are present. Without GSSG-to-GSH recycle and without antioxidant helpers, you cannot give enough GSH to get all of its responsibilities taken care of. With this understanding, here are some guidelines for GSH supplementation. Be sure to read the next part – adverse responses – before you give any supplemental GSH.

Years of Age	Milligrams of GSH/day, oral
Ages 2-4	50 to 150
Ages 5-10	100 to 250
Age 11 and above	100 to 300

A clinical study presented by Dr. Jill James at the October 2004 DAN! Conference showed the beneficial effects of betaine (TMG) and folinic acid on GSH levels in children with ASD (James SJ "Increased oxidative stress and impaired methylation capacity in children with autism: metabolic biomarkers and genetic predisposition" Fall DAN! Conference Proceedings, Los Angeles CA October 2004, 143-160). The TMG and folinic acid supplements increased cysteine and GSH levels and decreased the GSSG/GSH ratio significantly in a three-month intervention trial with 20 children. Total GSH was raised an average of 25% from baseline levels and the GSSG/GSH ratio was halved with daily supplements of TMG (1000 mg bid) and folinic acid (800 micrograms bid). So, in autism, attacking the biochemical problem of impaired methylation achieves another desired result – better glutathione levels – without having to give glutathione itself.

Adverse Response to Glutathione

You are supposed to use reduced, L-glutathione, GSH. Try to get some assurance from the provider or manufacturer that the product does not contain significant amounts of oxidized glutathione, GSSG. One percent GSSG is okay; five percent is not. Over time, some GSH users have developed intestinal overgrowth of yeast, especially Candida. Periodic or regular use of anti-yeast supplements is recommended: caprylic acid, olive leaf extract, goldenseal extract, perhaps Saccharomyces boulardii too.

If the ASD individual has any kind of insulin-dependent condition, consult your doctor before using supplements that contain glutathione. While small serving amounts of GSH are unlikely to cause insulin reduction, 100 mg quantities and above might do so.

Those with cystinuria (renal wasting of cystine) usually need GSH, but unfortunately GSH adds to cysteine supplies and formation of renal cystine stones are a risk with cystinuria. Again, low serving amounts usually are okay, higher amounts might not be.

About Glutathione (Optional Reading)

Reduced, active glutathione, GSH, is a tripeptide composed of glutamic acid, cysteine and glycine. The cysteinyl part (in the middle) carries a very reactive sulfhydryl part, -SH. Synthesis of GSH is magnesium-dependent; magnesium deficiency hinders the formation of GSH. The sulfhydryl group can trade its hydrogen for a bond or connection to atoms or molecules with affinity for sulfur. This allows GSH to connect with many unwanted substances and escort them out of the body, usually via bile and fecal matter. The give-away of hydrogen from the –SH part is an antioxidant function. Reducing hydrogen peroxide is an example of this:

$$\text{Peroxide} + 2\text{GSH} \xrightarrow{\text{GPx}} 2\text{H}_2\text{O} + \text{GSSG}$$

(Peroxide is changed into water, GSH gets oxidized.)

The enzyme that promotes this reaction, GPx, is glutathione peroxidase. The red blood cell version of GPx needs selenium for catalytic activity. This mechanism also works to protect lipids or fatty acids from oxidation, and it spares vitamin E from oxidation. Once GSSG is formed, it has to be rescued from its oxidized state and reduced back to its active GSH form. The enzyme that promotes this is glutathione reductase, GR. Although NADPH is the preferred reducing reactant, NADH will also do this.

$$GSSG + NADPH + H^+ \xrightarrow[\text{GR}]{} 2\,GSH + NADP^+$$

(Oxidized glutathione gets its hydrogen back, but then the cofactor form of niacin will need to get new hydrogen.)

Studies indicate that healthy mammals (including humans) maintain at least 98% of intracellular glutathione as GSH. Oxidant stress tends to increase the proportion of oxidized glutathione, GSSG. The supply of NADPH for GSSG recycle comes primarily from a part of human metabolism known as the "hexose monophosphate shunt", which uses sugar to drive the process.

Besides antioxidant work, GSH binds elements that might otherwise attach to and inactivate proteins, hormones and enzymes that contain sulfur. Metals that bind to GSH, roughly in order of decreasing affinity, are: mercury (Hg^{++}), free iron (Fe^{+++}), cadmium, nickel, copper, lead, cobalt, zinc and selenium. Mercury is reported to be escorted out of cells by GSH. However, if mercury gets free, it can exact revenge by poisoning the enzyme that promotes NADPH formation, thus impairing GSSG recycle to GSH.

Over the years, a controversy has festered over whether oral glutathione is beneficial. My opinion is a definite yes, at least for most individuals. Dietary GSH is absorbed into the bloodstream from the lumen of the small intestine. Not all dietary/oral GSH is digested. Research has demonstrated that direct, intact intestinal absorption of dietary GSH occurs as well as absorption via partial digestion followed by resynthesis in cells. How does GSH or a dipeptide piece of GSH survive digestion? It's because the cysteine in the middle is linked to the end of the glutamic part that's opposite to what our digestive enzymes are designed to handle. In other words, for durability, glutathione has its glutamic part on backwards.

Glutamic acid-cysteine-glycine = GSH (gamma-glutamyl-cysteinyl-glycine)

There's another controversial issue in GSH supplementation; it's about timing when a toxicant exposure is expected. It goes like this. Suppose you or your ASD loved one plans to eat seafood or shellfish that might contain mercury. Should you then simultaneously supplement GSH? My answer – No! Cysteine, GSH, NAC and other cysteinyl substances can carry toxicants like mercury into the bloodstream and make toxicant contamination worse. You want in-place, inside-tissue GSH to carry the bad stuff out. Or days later, you want supplemental GSH to go in, find the mercury and escort it out. You don't want to enhance the transport of incoming toxicants. So, if you expect or suspect a coming toxicant exposure, supplement beforehand and afterward, but not during.

Literature – Glutathione

Beutler E "Nutritional and metabolic aspects of glutathione" *Ann.Rev of Nutr*ition 9 (1989) 287-302

Meister A "Glutathione metabolism" in *Methods of Enzymology* 251 (1995) 3

Ormstad K and Orrenius S "Metabolism of extracellular glutathione in small intestine and kidney" in Glutathione: Storage, Transport and Turnover in Mammals, Sakamoto et al. eds. Japan Sci Soc Press (1983) 107-125

Bray TM and Taylor CG "Tissue glutathione, nutrition and oxidative stress" *Canadian J Physiol. Pharmacol* <u>71</u> (1993) 745-751

Mayes PA Chapt. 14 in Murray RK , Granner DK et al. eds <u>Harper's Biochemistry</u> 25th ed. Lange Med Pub (2000)

Vincenzini MT, Favilli F and Iantomasi T "Intestinal uptake and transmembrane transport systems of intact GSH; characteristics and possible biological role" *Biochimica et Biophysica Acta* <u>1113</u> (1992) 13-23

Hagen TM et al. "Fate of dietary glutathione: disposition in the gastrointestinal tract" *Am.Physiological Society*, 0193-1857-90 (1990) 6530-6535

Herbals

Except for Bacopa, there's only one general purpose in using herbals in ASD: to reduce inflammation. There are three actions that an herb can have that achieve this: (1) anti yeast/fungal, (2) antibacterial, (3) antioxidant or cytokine-lowering activity. Legally, nutritional supplement manufacturers can't make claims about some of this, especially actions (1) and (2). I'm not affiliated with any manufacturer or provider of supplements, so what follows is a brief synopsis of what I've learned. It's a short list of herbals because these are the ones that I know work and that don't cause problems if they are of good quality. There are hundreds of different herbals available in health food stores and from other sources, and each typically has lots of claims – often unsubstantiated. If you wish to try something I haven't described here, first investigate carefully and seek informed advice from a knowledgeable professional. Naturopathic doctors (N.D.s) are especially well-versed on the use of herbal products.

One almost-universal problem with herbals is assurance of purity. Foreign-source products, particularly, may be contaminated with toxicants or heavy metals. Be sure to deal with reputable sources.

For ease of use, all of these herbs are commercially available in capsule form. Since many of them have powerful flavors and aromas, you will want to use this form rather than trying to obtain and use the "bare" herb itself.

Anti-yeast/fungal substances (for use in Tier 2 and beyond)

Olive leaf extract, from the leaf of Olea europa, contains oleuropein (which helps keep the tree healthy), and this substance inhibits fungal growth. It's also antibacterial and it gives parasites a hard time. It's nontoxic at 100x the usually packaged "dose" per a pharmaceutical study (Upjohn, 1970). The effective daily amount is 200 to 400 mg in divided doses for a child 5 to 12 years old. Use less for younger children. I don't have feedback on adults but have no reason to think that 300 to, say, 600 mg wouldn't be beneficial in helping to control intestinal yeast overgrowth.

Pau d'Arco, also called Taheebo, is a tropical tree (Tabeluia avellanedae, also denoted as T. impetiginosa); the extract of the inner bark contains quinines that are antifungal and antibiotic. Useful daily amounts are similar to those of olive leaf extract: age 5 to 12, 200 to 400 mg/d; use less for younger children; 300 to 600 mg/d for older persons.

Oregano_is antifungal; see Antibacterial Herbals below for information about its major activity.

Goldenseal is antiyeast/fungal (candida primarily), see Antibacterial Herbals below for information about its major activity.

Not an herbal ,but powerfully anti-yeast/anti-fungal are **Saccharomyces boulardii** (see Probiotics) and the mid-chain-size fatty acid, **caprylic acid** or its calcium form, **calcium caprylate**. Caprylic acid is the fatty acid in our ear wax that inhibits yeast/fungal growth in our ear canals. 25 to 100 mg/d (orally) knocks out a lot of unwanted yeast. It's sold separately and as an ingredient in yeast-controlling formulations.

Antibacterial Herbals (for use in Tier 2 and beyond)

Oregano_comes from the perennial plant Origanum vulgare. Either the total herb or its oil fraction has powerful antibacterial action through several of its natural ingredients. If used for a period of weeks, the spore-formers (including Clostridia) are pretty much wiped out. Effective whole herb amounts range from 250 to 500 mg/d for age 5-12 years, less for younger children; 500 to 1000 mg/d for teens and adults. Sorry about the aroma. Even when encapsulated, it may not be to everyone's liking.

Thyme from the plant Thymus vulgaris also is a bacterial killer: Citrobacter, Clostridia, Proteus, Salmonella, and Staph aureus are some of its victims. Use the whole herb or oil fraction. Effective daily whole-herb amounts are the same as for oregano.

Goldenseal is Hydrastus canadensis, a perennial plant that grows in the woods in the Northeastern US and Canada. Its roots/rhizomes are yellowish (golden) and contain ber-berine and hydrastine; these are in the extract formulations. Goldenseal extract acts against E. coli, klebsiella, helicobacter and candida. Effective amounts are 100 to 200 mg/d for age 5-12, use less for younger children; 200 to 400 mg/d for teens and adults.

Antioxidant/Anti-inflammatory Herbals (Tier 1 and beyond)

Turmeric is the herb from the plant Curcuma longa and **curcumin** is a phytochemical component of turmeric. Turmeric is about the most powerful natural anti-inflammatory that you can use for an ASD individual. It lowers cytokine levels and it increases GSH lev-els in neurons and astrocytes (Lavoie S et al. *J. Neurochem* <u>108</u> (6) Mar 2009, 1410-22). This is exactly what we're looking for to help many with ASD. There are only two drawbacks – poor bioavailability and rapid removal from body tissues. This means we need to use a good amount several times per day: age 5 to 12, 200 mg, 3x per day, less for younger children; 200 to 400 mg, 3x per day for teens and adults. Allergic sensitivity is reported but uncommon.

Silymarin is a mixture of flavonoids extracted from the milk thistle plant Silybum marianum, sometimes called Mary's thistle. Milk thistle has been used medicinally since Pliny the Elder's writings in the first century AD, and its use could go back three or four centuries before that. Modern pharmacological studies document antioxidant and anti-inflammatory actions including destruction of free radicals and inhibition of lipid (fatty acid membrane) oxidation. Milk thistle extracts should contain 60 to 80% silymarin; effective amounts are: age 5 to 12 years, 50 to 100 mg 2x per day, less for younger children; 100 to 200 mg 3x per day for teens and adults.

Cognitive Improvement Herb – Bacopa

In spite of all the "get smarter, improve memory" hype on TV, the only one for which doctors claim some success is <u>Bacopa</u>, also called Brahmi; it comes from the plant Bacopa monniera. Its use originated in India and is documented back to the sixth century AD. Animal data show it to be a stimulator of GABA production in brain tissue; it allows rats/mice to more rapidly figure out and remember maze pathways. Controlled human studies accepted by scientists are lacking (Facts & Comparisons 2004), but doctors and parents have told me that it definitely helps their patients/children learn. Bacopa is packaged as powdered leaf and as powdered extract, where the extract should include "bacosides A and B". Suggested amounts are: ages 5 to 12 years, 20 to 40 mg/d of bacosides A and B, younger children may take 20 mg/d; teens and adults, 40 to 80 mg/d of bacosides A & B. Note that the leaf extract often is 20% bacosides A & B, so 100 mg of leaf extract provides the 20 mg of bacosides.

Literature – Herbals

Dorman HJD and Deans SG "Antimicrobial agents from plants: antibacterial activity of plant volatile oils" *J Appl Microbiol* 88 (2000) 308-316

Kulemba D and Kurnick A "Antibacterial and antifungal properties of essential oils" *Curr Med Chem* 10 (10) May 2003 813-29

Brennan M "Plant may hold key to ultimate antibiotic" *Chem Eng News*, Feb 21, 2000 6-7

Gao X et al "Immunomodulatory activity of curcumin…" *Biochem Pharmacol* 68 (1) Jul 2, 2004, 51-61

Yadav VS et al. "Immunomodulatory effects of curcumin" *Immunopharmacol Immunotoxicol* 27 (3) 2005, 485-97

Bengmark S "Curcumin, an atoxic antioxidant and natural NFkappaB, cyclooxygenase-2, lipooxygenase and induceable nitric oxide inhibitor…" *J Parenteral Enteral Nutr* 30 (1) Jan-Feb 2006, 45-51.

Melatonin

This is a hormone-like substance that the body makes from serotonin, which comes from an essential amino acid, tryptophan. Many parents of autistic children have reported that just one or two milligrams each evening have helped sleep and behavior. Melatonin has the best parent-response score for any single, oral nutritional supplement (66% reported improved behaviors).

Indications of Need

These include poor sleep or disordered sleep patterns, crying at night, circadian dysrhythm, persistent signs of oxidant stress or inflammation. If serotonin also is deficient, there can be extra sensitivity to light and sound, food cravings with lack of satiety, and anxiety. Consistent with insufficient melatonin are diagnoses of tryptophan deficiency (by amino acid analysis), Hartnup disorder (malabsorption of tryptophan leading to toxicants produced by intestinal flora), intestinal dysbiosis (esp. clostridia), vitamin B_6 deficiency or

P5P coenzyme dysfunction, biopterin deficiency, impaired SAM methylation or elevated adenosine or elevated adenosylhomocysteine/SAM ratio. Elevated inflammation markers (cytokines) are consistent as well.

When and how much?

I have found, as many others have, that the effective daily amount of supplemental melatonin is quite variable from one individual to another. Usually one or two milligrams given about one hour before bedtime works well, but for a few, half a milligram does the trick. Others may need up to five milligrams, but this is unusual. Often, trial-and-error is needed to decide on the best amount, and two or three nights should be the trial period for each amount. Time-release melatonin supplements became available a few years ago; I suggest that these be given a try. Often, a two-milligram time-release tablet does wonders for sleep and behavior. If you do try the time-release type, do not break, crush or dissolve the tablet before giving it – that ruins the time-release chemistry.

Adverse Response to Melatonin?

As of 2009, the ARI parent Response Tally (ARI Publication 34) showed the following for melatonin, 1687 parents reporting –

Behavior or Traits Improved	No Discernible Effect	Behavior or Traits Worsened
66%	26%	8%

Melatonin's actions depend greatly on amount and on sensory inputs, especially light and perhaps sound. For it to work, you will have to keep the child's bedroom dark and quiet. Parent reports and published science indicate that once the child's eyes open to light, an internal switch occurs. The body then seems to assume that melatonin's night work is done, release by the pineal gland stops, and catabolism (destruction) of the melatonin begins. (For those with chemistry and physiology interest, melatonin is hydroxylated and then either sulfated or glucuronidated and expelled in urine.)

Melatonin's actions can also be cut short if too much is present. This also seems to throw the stop-releasing-and-get-rid-of-it switch. So, using too much can produce an effect opposite of what's desired.

If your child's sleep patterns aren't improved after giving melatonin a good try, be sure you're giving taurine. You should be doing that, because it's a Tier 1 supplement, too. If melatonin doesn't help at this time, you may have to wait until other measures correct disordered adenosine metabolism, possibly as far along as Tiers 4 or 5. Be sure that digestion and diet have been looked after. Nobody sleeps well with indigestion. Also, high-protein meals before bedtime can seriously impair tryptophan passage into the brain and limit synthesis of serotonin and melatonin.

About Melatonin (and Serotonin and Tryptophan, Optional)

The neurohormone melatonin is is made in the pineal gland from serotonin. (A neurohormone is a natural body chemical that signals the nervous system to do something.) The formation process for melatonin starts with a nutritionally essential amino acid, tryptophan; it progresses to serotonin (a hormone and neurotransmitter) and then moves on to melatonin.

Dietary tryptophan is obtained by digestion of protein foods: legumes such as peanuts, peas and soy protein; turkey, chicken and eggs; beef and fish. Most tryptophan is used outside the brain and CNS to form products such as serotonin, nicotinic acid (form of vitamin B_3), picolinate and the amino acid alanine. If dietary protein is not completely digested or if there is malabsorption of tryptophan for any reason, the consequences are not good for autism or ASD. Dysbiotic flora, especially the clostridia genus of bacteria, like to consume tryptophan, and they produce somewhat toxic chemicals from it. The take-home lesson is that giving tryptophan to increase serotonin and melatonin or to improve mood, sleep, eating habits, etc. can be perilous in autism. A tryptophan supplement (by doctor's recommendation) may be okay if there's no tryptophan malabsorption problem and there's no bacterial dysbiosis (esp. clostridia). Tryptophan requires biopterin and vitamin B_6 as P5P to become serotonin, so vitamin B_6 adequacy is another requirement for formation of serotonin and melatonin.

Years ago, pure L-tryptophan became available in health food stores and from manufacturers of nutritional supplements. Following illness attributed to a contaminated batch of tryptophan manufactured in Japan, the FDA in 1988 recalled all nutritional products that contained manufactured tryptophan. Foods or supplements that contain tryptophan naturally were not included in the recall. Then, following several legal challenges, the FDA in 2001 issued a statement relaxing the ban to some degree. Importation of foreign-manufactured tryptophan remains illegal, and manufacturers are solely responsible for tryptophan purity and safety. Today, tryptophan is again available as a supplement from some mail-order suppliers and at some health food stores.

In abdominal tissues, serotonin can act as a vasoconstrictor. If, for example, toxicant uptake is occurring from the intestines via capillary blood vessels, serotonin might be produced in relatively large quantities to restrict capillary flow. Serotonin also can restrict release of digestive juices by the stomach and it's also a regulator of lactation.

It is reported that some with ASD (perhaps 20%) have elevated blood serotonin while others (5%?) have been reported as low. The measured specimen for serotonin in these cases is whole blood or blood platelets, or, in a few cases, serum. Most published reports are for whole blood serotonin, with about one in five elevated. I tend to connect that finding with vasoconstrictor function in capillaries in and around intestinal tissue. The assumed reason is to reduce toxicant uptake – but that is just my opinion. If blood serotonin is measured as low, the sensible thing to do next would be to measure blood plasma tryptophan level (maybe it's low too?). In clinical research on ASD, this analytical followup of measuring tryptophan and serotonin levels and also measuring the products of serotonin metabolism has been woefully incomplete. What's needed is a comprehensive picture of the tryptophan-serotonin-melatonin family, including metabolic daughter products.

Perhaps the most important aspect of serotonin is that measured blood levels might or might not reflect brain and CNS levels. Serotonin itself does not cross an intact blood-brain barrier. Tryptophan does cross and is the starting material for synthesis of brain serotonin and melatonin. If dietary uptake of tryptophan is limited and if blood serotonin is high, there's a chance that brain tryptophan, serotonin and melatonin could be low. So, blood levels of these substances do not necessarily reflect brain levels, and brain levels could be opposite from what blood indicates.

Another problem with tryptophan is transport into the brain when it has competition. Tryptophan is about the least abundant amino acid – least abundant in food proteins, least abundant in human protein and least abundant in many body tissues and fluids. Tryptophan is especially vulnerable to being crowded out of blood-brain transit by other amino acids. Histidine, phenylalanine, tyrosine, valine and leucine at moderate-to-high levels in blood can impede tryptophan's ability to get into the brain. In other words, eating a large portion of high-protein food for supper is not conducive to getting tryptophan into the brain. When this happens, lowered levels of serotonin and melatonin and poor quality sleep are likely outcomes.

Besides the pineal gland, serotonin is stored in tiny sacs at the end of nerve cells (neurons). Reacting to an electrical impulse (neuronal activity and information transport), serotonin is released from the sac into the synapse – the space between two neurons. It then has neurotransmitter activity. When the serotonin finds and binds to receptors on the adjacent cell, it produces an inhibitory influence on neuronal activity. This has a calming or soothing effect and results in feelings of contentment. When serotonin is deficient, there is increased perception of sensory signals, alertness, uneasiness and maybe even anxiety. Serotonin is not available as a nutritional supplement, and even if it were, it wouldn't do much good for mood control because it doesn't cross into the brain from the blood.

For normal humans, the rate-limiting step of melatonin formation is activation (acetylation) of serotonin. This is a chemical prerequisite to methylation, the final step in melatonin assembly. For most acetylation, our bodies use a rather large, reactive agent, acetyl-coenzyme A. (Please refer to pantothenic acid in the Vitamins chapter for more information on Coenzyme A.) For many of those with autism, I believe the final step, methylation, is the problem. SAM (S-adenosylmethionine) has to donate its methyl group to acetylated serotonin to form melatonin. Clinical and analytical studies by Professor Richard Deth (Northeastern University), Dr. S. Jill James (Arkansas Children's Hospital) and others show that a significant portion of the ASD population has trouble with SAM methylation. My conviction about this is that at least 40% of tested but untreated ASD individuals have impaired SAM methylation. And then there's the deciding factor – the 66% of 1687 individuals who are reported by parents to have improved with a melatonin supplement. (ARI Pub.34, 2009)

The bottom line is that a melatonin supplement is the best trial intervention for disordered sleep patterns and for the other, previously-listed indications – at least early on. Until digestion is working, with a friendly gut flora environment and metabolism in good order, tryptophan use is too risky.

Below is some additional information on melatonin with references for those who would like to learn more about the single most successful single nutrient supplement for autistic individuals.

Melatonin is considered to be a regulator of human circadian rhythm. It can induce sleep when other influences for sleep are inadequate. Melatonin can cause sleep and wakefulness phase shifts in the body's daily clock. This has led to the concept of using melatonin to counter insomnia. One possible mechanism for this is sensitization of adenylate cyclase, which melatonin does in certain cells of the pituitary gland. Cellular perception often depends upon adenylate cyclase which is an enzyme that participates in message processing by cells. Melatonin also is reported to influence tissue and organ activity via G-protein-coupled receptors. See Guanosine in Glossary.)

There is also a report that melatonin upregulates the enzyme pyridoxal kinase in brain tissue. This is the enzyme that promotes phosphate addition and forms pyridoxal phosphate or pyridoxine phosphate from pyridoxal or pyridoxine. Pyridoxal 5-phosphate is the active coenzyme form of vitamin B_6. Phosphorylation of pyridoxine is the step that Dr. Tapan Audhya did analytical studies of, and found to be very slow in autistics.

Finally, there are literature reports of antioxidant and anti-cytokine activity of melatonin. A cytokine is a protein or peptide that is released from inflamed tissue. Tumor-necrosis-factor alpha ($TNF\alpha$) is a cytokine that may be elevated in autism. $TNF\alpha$ may cause decreased sulfation capability. Melatonin helps to regulate the expression of antioxidant enzyme genes. It protects against lipid peroxidation by hydrogen peroxide, and it scavenges the hydroxyl radical (as does vitamin C), which means that melatonin helps to protect DNA from oxidant attack. Melatonin is considered by some to be an antioxidant vitamin. Of course, it's a vitamin only to those who cannot make enough of it in their own bodies, and this group appears to include a majority of those on the autistic spectrum.

Literature - Melatonin

PDA for Nutritional Supplements, Thomson PDR, 1st Ed (2001) p .301-06

Baker SM and K Baar The Circadian Prescription, GP Putnam & Sons (2000)

Gillberg C and M Coleman The Biology of the Autistic Syndromes, 2nd Edition, MacKeith Press (1992), Chapter 10, p. 115-130

Babal K "The Fall and Rise of Tryptophan" Nutr Sci News 3 no.2 (Feb 1998) 60-64

Lincoln GA, H Andersen and D Hazelrigg "Clock genes and the long-term regulation of prolactin secretion…" J Neuroendocrinology 15 no.4 (2003) 390-397

Barrett P, C Schuister et al. "Sensitization: a mechanism for melatonin action in the pars tuberalis" J.Neuroendocrinology 15 no.4 (2003) 415-421

Johnson JD et al. "Gonadotrophin-releasing hormone drives melatonin receptor…" Proceedings, Nat.Acad.Sci (USA) 100 no.5 (2003) 2831-2835

Saski M et al. "Melatonin reduces $TNF\alpha$ induced expression of MAdCAM-1 via inhibition of NF-Kappa B" Brit Med.Coll Gastroenterology 2 no.1 (2002)9

Mayo JC et al. "Melatonin regulation of antioxidant enzyme gene expression" Cell Mol Life Sci 59 no.10 (2002) 1706-1713

Tan DX et al. "Melatonin, a hormone, a tissue factor, a paracoid and an antioxicant vitamin" J.Pineal Research 34 no.1 (2003) 75-78

~Introduction to Elements and Minerals~

Calcium in more or less pure chemical form is an element. It's a metal that you've probably never seen, because it's extremely reactive – meaning it combines readily and rapidly with other elements. When it does, some of these combinations are called minerals, especially those we find in nature. Calcium carbonate (calcite) and calcium phosphate (apatite) are mineralized forms of calcium. The former exists in the earth as limestone and the latter (as hydroxyapatite) is a major part of animal and human bone structure. In nutrition, we tend to use the words mineral and element interchangeably, but to a chemist, there's a big difference.

Essentially, our bodies are composed of about two dozen elements in many chemical forms. Some of these elements are understood to be necessary for life but they are traditionally omitted from the list of nutritionally essential elements – carbon, oxygen, hydrogen, sulfur and chlorine. Then, there is a group of elements that physiologists and nutritionists have argued about in terms of physiologic need – lithium, boron, fluorine, silicon and vanadium. And then, there are the ones that are traditionally listed as nutritionally essential minerals. These thirteen elements with their chemical shorthand symbols are:

Calcium	Ca	Molybdenum	Mo
Chromium	Cr	Phosphorus	P
Copper	Cu	Potassium	K
Iodine	I	Selenium	Se
Iron	Fe	Sodium	Na
Magnesium	Mg	Zinc	Zn
Manganese	Mn		

Five of these essentials (Ca, Mg, I, Se and Zn) plus sulfur are of concern in autism and ASD. Before we discuss these, I'd like to take issue with the commonly recited, orthodox dictum: "If you eat a healthy diet, you don't need vitamin and mineral supplements." I'm directing this at you, reader – you personally. This goes way beyond the scope of what supplement might benefit someone with ASD.

The USDA and university food research teams measured the mineral (element) content of foods decades ago, mostly before World War II. Since WWII, much of our farmland has been in constant use with chemical fertilization applied to bolster annual growth of crops. Nitrogen and ammonia, potassium (potash), phosphorus, and a couple of other minerals are provided by the fertilizers. As a rule, I haven't seen soil replenishment of copper, zinc, selenium, manganese, molybdenum, etc. – have you?

I think it was in the fall of 1992 that I was sitting at my work desk in Doctor's Data Laboratory (then in West Chicago, IL). My associate, Bob Smith, showed up with two grocery bags full of fruits and vegetables. At that time, I was president of Doctor's Data Lab and Bob ("Mister Hair Analysis") was Vice President of Doctor's Data, Inc.

The grocery bags were labeled "A" and "B". That's all I knew, except that each contained apples, pears, potatoes, whole wheat flour, wheat berries, and sweet corn. "Please analyze these for all the elements, nutritional, toxic and otherwise that our instrument can accurately measure" was his request. You would have had to know Bob to not be surprised by his asking this in a clinical laboratory that measures and reports on what's in blood plasma, cells, urine, hair, etc. The month before, it was shark blood from Sea World, and before that it was flesh from farmed salmon. I shrugged and said, "Sure, but it won't happen until next Friday." Bob, of course, expected more immediate attention to his latest project, but I had people samples in line ahead of groceries.

A week later, I had the results. Here are a few of them, presented as Bob wanted – elemental contents of produce in bag B as a percentage, higher or lower, of those in bag A. In other words, bag A contained reference produce, and how is the stuff in bag B different?

Apples in Bag B	Less than Bag A	More than Bag A
Calcium		40%
Magnesium		40%
Manganese		50%
Phosphorus		75%
Mercury	90%	
Wheat in Bag B		
Calcium		120%
Magnesium		430%
Manganese		540%
Phosphorus		240%
Mercury	40%	
Corn in Bag B		
Calcium		1800%
Magnesium		300%
Manganese		1600%
Phosphorus		210%
Mercury		80%

"So, Bob, what's Bag A and what's Bag B?", I asked. "Bag A, he said, was food I bought at the supermarket – regular, commercial produce. Bag B contains all organic foods."

The entire report on this, for 26 measured elements in organic foods versus regular commercial (supermarket) foods, is published – Smith, BL, "Organic Foods vs Supermarket Foods: Element Levels" *Journal of Applied Nutrition*, vol. 45, no. 1, 1993, p. 35-39.

You might ask why the mercury went up in organic corn vs the commercial type. Actually, commercial corn was very low in mineral content, and the percentage increase in mercury was due to a very tiny amount of increase over a very tiny amount in the commercial product.

The moral to the story is that, unless you're regularly eating good quality organic foods, you're probably not getting the amounts of essential minerals that books indicate or that the medical establishment believes to exist in our food. Just think, ounce for ounce, the tested organic wheat contained 430% more magnesium than did the supermarket brand. That's why supplements can help most people – a lot!

Calcium, Ca

For people with ASD, findings of subnormal calcium levels have been occasional and mostly by urine or hair element analyses. With normal dietary intake of calcium, a finding of low urine levels implies subnormal uptake or malabsorption. Over 30 years ago, calcium was found to be low in autistic children with celiac disease or with a history of colic. Since then, low or marginal calcium levels per hair or urine analysis have been observed from time to time at higher frequencies than in the normal population. I've conjectured that poor digestion, including fat malabsorption, is part of the mechanism that limits uptake of dietary calcium. Calcium status does not show well in blood, where it can be deceptively normal even in gross calcium disorders such as osteoporosis. And hair calcium levels can be high and deceptive when calcium metabolism is disturbed. Admittedly, hair is a lousy tissue for calcium assessment and I mention it only because it has been used a lot.

With ASD, calcium adequacy is a common concern when a casein-free diet is tried or instituted. Such diets eliminate milk and dairy products and thus reduce dietary calcium by a significant amount. (For a typical child in the US, cows' milk provides up to 75% of total dietary calcium.)

Indications of Need

Need for a calcium supplement is virtually certain for children and most adults on a casein-free diet. Other indications include laboratory test results with medical/nutritional input. While blood and cell elemental analyses which include calcium assay are offered by a number of clinical laboratories, "normal" results on such tests often are deceiving. Most cells do not contain much calcium inside, and blood transport of calcium doesn't reflect body stores. Bone density does, but it's a rather late indicator of calcium deficiency. Deficient vitamin D by analytical test usually means calcium is low too, and low magnesium in blood cells or serum is a suspicious condition in which calcium might also be low. Other conditions consistent with insufficient calcium uptake include: digestive deficiency/disorder, fat malabsorption, steatorrhea, oxalate excess, parathyroid dysfunction, low-protein diet, muscle cramps, and deficiency of acidophilic flora (e.g. Lactobacillus acidophilus) in the intestinal tract. L. acidophilus optimizes the intestinal pH for best uptake of calcium. Sometimes hyperactivity is due to calcium deficiency.

About half of ASD children are measured to have increased fat in their stools (per lab analysis –Jeffrey Bradstreet, MD, ARI/DAN! Conference, Atlanta, 2001). That corresponds to increased fat in the intestines – unabsorbed dietary fat. While less severe than that of a steatorrhea diagnosis, increased intestinal fat means less calcium is available for assimilation into the bloodstream. It also means that oxalic acid in foods forms less calcium oxalate in the intestines. That, in turn, means more oxalic acid uptake and more oxalate inside the body (not good). Use of a digestive enzyme supplement that includes lipase may significantly increase uptake of dietary fats and calcium in many with ASD.

When and How Much?

Below, I've tabulated the calcium needs of children to provide an idea of how much alternative-source calcium is required when dairy is excluded from the diet, assuming dairy provides 75% of need.

Age (years)	Weight (lbs) Nominal	Calcium RDA, mg/d*	mg/d needed in substitute food or supplements if milk is excluded
0.5-1	20	800	600
1-2	29	800	600
4-6	44	800	600
7-10	62	1200	900
11-14	99	1200	900

*The FDA daily serving (supplement label) is 1000 mg calcium per day. Up to 1200 is recommended by the Institute of Medicine, Food and Nutrition Board of the National Academy of Science

Part of the calcium that makes up for excluding milk from the diet can be in nutritional supplement form. Another part may be provided by drinks that substitute for cows' milk, such as rice milk, soy milk (if tolerated), "milk" made from nuts, etc. You'll need to know how much calcium is in the substitute foods to figure out how much supplemental calcium you need to add. Ask your nutrition counselor for help on this.

Depending on the amount needed, the best times to supplement calcium in order of preference are: supper, lunch, breakfast. Don't do large amounts at one time; split the daily total up if possible, such as supper 300 mg, lunch 200 mg, breakfast, 100 mg. Calcium often has a calming effect, and calming before nighttime is a definite benefit.

Is calcium carbonate a good form for an autistic person to use? (Carbonate may include eggshells and coral forms.) Yes, provided that it is combined with another, more soluble, form, and provided that lead contamination is insignificant. Using two or more forms of calcium evens out the absorption period for uptake from the gastrointestinal tract.

The advantage of calcium carbonate is its calcium content – it's 40% calcium by weight versus about 20% for most citrates, and less than 10% for most organic salts such as gluconate. If your child needs 200 mg of supplemental calcium, that's 500 mg of calcium carbonate (one big capsule or maybe two smaller ones), or 1000 mg of citrate (maybe four capsules), or over 2000 mg of gluconate (lots of capsules).

Is all calcium citrate a good idea? For you and me, it's probably fine. For an individual with ASD, all Ca citrate isn't such a good idea. Citrate is not completely processed in many autistics, and urine organic acid tests frequently show higher than normal amounts of excreted citrate. This may be secondary to several physiological problems: decreased output of bicarbonate by a malfunctioning pancreas, decreased capability of citric acid-processing enzymes, and possibly interference with the citric acid cycle by mimic compounds from dysbiotic gut flora. The citric acid cycle is a mitochondrial process; please refer to the Glossary if you wish to know more about this.

Is calcium lactate a good idea? Calcium lactate is a calcium salt of lactic acid (not the sugar lactose). As with citrate, urine organic acid tests for autistics have shown elevated lactate, but this occurs less often than elevated citrate does. And, for that matter, pyruvate may also be elevated. Pyruvate, lactate and citrate are all clustered near the same place metabolically, and that place seems to present problems for many autistics. So, I'd avoid lactate supplements unless I knew from analytical testing that it would be okay for the individual. Calcium lactate is nominally 18% calcium. 100 milligrams of calcium corresponds to 455 milligrams of lactate.

Can I count the calcium that's in calcium ascorbate as part of the calcium supplement? You can count only about one third of it. Up to two thirds is going to come out in the urine as a companion ion to dehydroascorbate and unused ascorbate, depending upon magnesium status. With plentiful magnesium, less calcium is wasted (at the expense of magnesium).

Should vitamin D be in the calcium supplement? Yes, or it should be in companion supplements. The same 5 year old child who needs 800 mg/d of calcium also needs 400 IU of vitamin D per day.

Other supplemental forms of calcium –

Amino acid chelates such as calcium glycinate: generally well tolerated, have excellent solubility and bioavailability regardless of stomach acidity. They also have a purity advantage.

Hydroxyapatite: use purified or synthetic forms as natural-bone forms sometimes have lead or strontium impurities; occasionally even uranium. Excellent supplemental form when pure; contains phosphate in the natural bone-matrix amount. Not as bioavailable as glycinate.

Gluconate: okay, good bioavailablity, but has low calcium content.

Phosphates: marginal as a calcium replenisher. The problem with it is the large amount of phosphate that can attach to other nutrients, like zinc, and make them less bioavailable. For calcium plus phosphate, go with hydroxyapatite.

Sulfate: okay only in small amounts (<25mg per serving). Very limited tolerance to larger oral amounts.

Caseinate: No! this is a calcium salt of casein.

Adverse response to Calcium Supplements?

ARI Publication 34, 2009 edition, shows only 3% with adverse responses to calcium supplements, n=2832. My experience in working with parents and doctors on this is that there is usually one of two possible problems. One – too much is being given at one time and maybe at the wrong time of day. Two – a calcium form is being used that isn't well tolerated. As mentioned above, try to split up the total daily calcium supplement with P.M. emphasis in amount, and give it with food. Sometimes using two different forms of calcium works best. There are occasional problems with calcium citrate and calcium lactate, possibly due to too much citrate or lactic acid already present. A urine test for organic acid levels tells the tale on whether there are hang-ups in metabolism of either of these.

There will be a problem if lots of calcium is given at the same time that zinc is given. Some of the zinc won't get absorbed. Give the zinc about two hours after the evening meal and then the suppertime calcium won't interfere with it.

Calcium glycinate is a common ingredient in high-quality calcium supplements, but it too can be troublesome for some people, especially if glycine is contained in their other supplements. When glycine metabolism is disordered, some of it becomes glyoxalate and some of that becomes oxalate in body tissues. It is hard to say how much supplemental glycine is too much when oxalate is excessive, but I'd start to be concerned when supplemented glycine exceeds 1000 mg/d for someone with oxalate excess. This problem can occur if vitamin B_6 as P5P has deficient activity, or if methylene THF is deficient (see folate chapter). Hyperoxaluria (high urine oxalate) means too much internal oxalate. Sometimes this happens genetically, and vitamin supplements don't help enough. Sometimes the real problem is fat malabsorption due to lipase insufficiency (as mentioned above). An additional strategy is use of taurine, which can bolster formation of bile, and that's important for absorbing fat-soluble nutrients (including vitamin D). Usually the oxalate problem then goes away and calcium assimilation improves.

While much has been said about oxalate and autism, we shouldn't exaggerate the issue. But if you've tested the individual for oxalate (in urine), and you're using a vitamin supplement that contains B_6 and folate, and you're using lipase in the digestive enzyme supplement, and taurine is being supplemented, and oxalate still is high, then reduce total supplemental glycine – not just calcium glycinate. If you do test for oxalates, be very sure the sample is processed promptly. The longer urine sits, the more it can change and the higher the oxalate content may be. You want a result that represents the patient, not the time on the lab bench.

Iodine, I, and Thyroid Support

The nutritionally essential element iodine is used exclusively for formation of thyroid hormones. Historically, tests of thyroid function in sample autistic populations did not conclude that iodine or thyroid hormone needed to be supplemented. There were, however, individuals who did show clinical improvement with thyroid hormone supplements. If the ASD person in your life needs nutritional support from supplemental iodine, or needs thyroid hormone supplementation, then that is a requirement which has to be met before you can expect significant improvement in other areas, including, surprisingly, development of healthy intestinal flora.

Indications of Need

- Abnormal thyroid test results involving TSH, T_3, T_4 as ordered and interpreted by your doctor
- Subnormal basal body temperature (consult your doctor)
- Periodic regrowth of intestinal yeast despite various anti-yeast measures
- Low iodine according to hair element analysis (hair is a valid tissue for assessing iodine status)
- Living in an area known to be contaminated with perchlorate, or living near a military base where solid-fuel rockets have been fired. If you are uncertain about this, I suggest an online search to determine if you live in or near one of the hundreds of locations where perchlorate contamination has been found in water, soil or food crops.

When and How Much?

If a hypothyroid condition exists, then primary treatment is prescribed by your doctor; it probably will be hormone supplementation rather than iodine supplements. If lithium is used by prescription at pharmacologic doses, consult your doctor before using an iodine supplement. The standard form for supplemental iodine is potassium iodide; I don't know of any reasons to use a different form. Too much is just as bad as not enough, so it's best to seek nutritional advice before using it. The daily serving or recommended amounts of dietary iodine are:

Age	Micrograms (mcg)
6 mos – 1 yr	50
1-6 yrs (WHO)	90
7-12 yrs (WHO)	120
1-10 yrs (FDA)	70 to 120
Over 11 yrs (FDA)	120 to 150
Pregnancy	175
Lactation	200

The US FDA daily serving (supplement label) amount is 150 mcg.

Adverse Response to Iodine?

Autoimmune thyroiditis and cystic fibrosis can be contraindicating conditions for iodine supplements. Symptoms of iodine overdose include acne flare-ups, skin rash, numbness and tingling in hands and feet, and headache. I very strongly favor use of multivitamin/multimineral supplements that have iodine as an included ingredient, over stand-alone iodine supplements.

Be absolutely sure that the quantities to be supplemented are micrograms (mcg) and **not** milligrams (mg). I've seen too many mistakes in talks and presentations on this point.

About Iodine and Perchlorate (Optional Reading)

In the US, the amount of iodine consumed in food can vary from less than a hundred micrograms up to more than a milligram per day. In countries where seafood is a staple of the diet, total daily intake may reach 10 or 20 mg, as they do in Japan. Unneeded iodine leaves by fecal matter. If it's absorbed, a further unneeded portion is excreted in urine. In the US, we consider the daily need in food to be 150 mcg, and textbooks tell us that about 50 mcg (one-third) of this goes to thyroglobulin formation.

Using the amino acid tyrosine, the body adds iodine atoms successively until, with two joined tyrosine parts, it has made throxine or T_4. The completed molecule holds four iodine atoms. This is primarily a reserve or storage form of the hormone; the active form is T_3, "triiodothronine". T_3 is made enzymatically from T_4 prohormone with an enzyme that's activated by selenium – a fact not discovered until 1990. So, thyroid function really depends upon adequacy of two nutritionally essential elements, iodine and selenium.

For years, doctors told me that patients, including those with autistic traits, develop and redevelop intestinal yeast overgrowth if they have subnormal thyroid function ("hypothyroid"). I would nod respectfully, always wondering why. Some doctors postulated reduced ability to mount adequate immune response. Finally, one day I ran across a much more intriguing fact about thyroxine, the prohormone. It mediates absorption of glucose from the intestine. Not enough thyroid hormone means sugar is left in the intestines for yeast to feed and grow on.

Until recently, there was little evidence of iodine insufficiency or subnormal thyroid function in children or adults with autism. In their book, *The Biology of the Autistic Syndromes* (Prager, 1985), Drs. Coleman and Gillberg review the pertinent clinical studies on thyroid function that were performed during 1950s through 1980. In all cases, the general finding was normal thyroid function or "euthroid" condition for the autistic subjects. Despite this, there were occasional reports of improved clinical condition when the hormone was administered. However, confirmation of benefit from thyroxine use in subsequent, carefully controlled studies, did not support an outcome of general improvement. (This probably is yet another example showing that we shouldn't average clinical results for ASD populations.)

In 2006, Professor James Adams (Arizona State University) and colleagues published a hair element analysis study of 51 ASD children, 29 mothers of ASD children, 40 neurotypical control children, and 25 mothers of the control children. Hair iodine levels were down by an average of 45% (statistically significant, $p = 0.005$) in the group of ASD children (3-15 years of age).

Again, this is a study that averaged the results; some of the ASD children may have had normal hair iodine, some levels down a little bit, and some down a lot. This study is published as: Adams JB, Holloway CE, et al. "Analysis of Toxic Metals and Essential Minerals in the Hair of Arizona Children with Autism and Associated Conditions and Their Mothers" *Bio Trace Element Res* 110 (2006) 193-209; Humana Press Inc.

The mothers of the ASD children had somewhat higher hair iodine levels than did the mothers of the control children (averaged). So, the iodine's available to the family, but the ASD children were assimilating much less of it per the hair test. And hair iodine does not directly translate to thyroid function. Hair is a screening test and therapeutic intervention should not be based on it alone. But low iodine in hair is a valid reason for a doctor to do further tests of thyroid hormones and function.

What changed between the 1950s-80s and 2006? For one thing, perchlorate happened. Perchlorate is a solid chemical that provides oxygen for solid-fueled rocket propulsion. Leakages from manufacturing facilities, plant explosions and military use caused perchlorate contamination of ground water and food supply in 22 states (*Chemical &Engineering News*, August, 2003). Perchlorate interferes with biological uptake of iodine. In other words, the food supply of iodine is probably as it always was, but due to perchlorate, assimilation of iodine, and consequently thyroxine formation, can be depressed. So, it's possible that iodine and thyroid status weren't an issue in ASD until the 1990s when environmental contamination became significant.

Ammonium perchlorate manufacture for military use began in 1951. Two plants were manufacturing the chemical in the 1980s, and one of them blew up in 1988 (PEPCON, Henderson, Nevada). In 1997 the replacement perchlorate plant blew up, too. It was in Utah. The problem is that agriculture (growing vegetables) in southern California uses Colorado River water whose watershed got the perchlorate contamination from the Nevada explosion. And the problem of military use of perchlorate goes all the way east to the Massachusetts Military Reservation on Cape Cod. How long is this environmental mess going to last? An exposé on it was published in *Chemical and Engineering News*, August 18, 2003, pages 37-46, and the answer to the question is an estimated 24 years (J. Batusta, Professor of Environmental Engineering, UNLV).

If you haven't already done so, you might have your ASD loved one checked for thyroid function. Chris and I did, and our son was diagnosed as hypothyroid by doctors at the University of Chicago Medical Center. He was put on a daily thyroid supplement. If thyroid function is depressed, then a thyroid hormone supplement is a lot better than just supplemental iodine.

Magnesium, Mg

Magnesium deficiency occurs in ASD for several reasons, one of which is urinary loss. This happens when taurine is deficient (see chapter on taurine) and may also occur following toxicant exposures.

Indications of Need

Analytically, need is determined by laboratory assay of element levels in blood cells (most valid), also in plasma or serum. Urine element tests can be deceptive because of urinary wasting of magnesium. There are published "magnesium loading tests" that your doctor might know or can read about.

1. Seelig C <u>Magnesium Deficiency in the Pathogenesis of Disease</u> Plenum Press NY, 1980, 367-69
2. Seelig C "Magnesium Deficiency" *Southern Med Journal* <u>83</u> no.7, July 1990 739-42
3. Holl M, Baker S. "Magnesium status as determined by retention of an intramuscular magnesium load: Repletion and monitoring of symptoms" *J Am Diet Assn* 1990; suppl. 90:37
4. Baker SM "Magnesium in Primary Care and Preventive Medicine: Clinical Correlation of Magnesium Loading Studies" *Magnes Trace Elem* 1991-92:251-262

Symptoms consistent with magnesium insufficiency include –

- Muscle twitches, sometimes confused with the "tics" of Gilles de la Tourette's Syndrome
- Constipation
- Muscle cramps, "tight" muscles
- Anxiety, panic attacks
- Insomnia
- Limited physical endurance
- Numbness or tingling in fingers, hands, toes, feet
- Multiple chemical sensitivities, inflammation

What Kind, When, and How Much?

If lithium is used by prescription, consult your doctor before using a magnesium supplement. It is good practice to provide a magnesium supplement when vitamin B_6 is used. If there's already magnesium in the vitamin formulation, then you may not need a separate, additional supplement unless lab tests indicate so or symptoms of need persist. See the vitamin chapter for matching magnesium amounts to vitamin B_6 supplements.

As an oral nutritional supplement, magnesium is available as amino acid chelates, such as glycinate chelate, as oxide (buffered), and as salts of aspartate, malate, and gluconate. Magnesium malate can be especially beneficial for ASD. Liquid supplements may contain magnesium as the chloride or sulfate, and these are very bioavailable forms.

The best time for a separate magnesium supplement is with calcium at the evening meal. Like calcium, it usually has a calming effect.

Many trials of magnesium for autistic individuals have been carried out by parents and doctors. From these trials, we learn that the effective Mg supplementation range is 3 milligrams to 8 milligrams per kilogram of body weight per day (or 1.5 mg to 4 mg per pound of body weight per day). For a 25-Kg (55 lb) four to six year old, for example, this is 80 to 220 mg/d of a magnesium in a supplement of some form. An initial low-dose trial of magnesium would be 0.5 to 1.0 mg/Lb of body weight (1 to 2 mg per kilogram) and not more than 100 mg in any case. The adult RDI or "Daily Value" for magnesium is 400 milligrams per day (mg/d).

Adverse Response to Magnesium Supplements?

According to the March 2009 edition of ARI Publication 34, there have been 301 parent responses to use of just magnesium (not included are the B_6 + magnesium responses).

Behavior or Traits Improved	No Discernible Effect	Behavior or Traits Worsened
29%	65%	6%

The most commonly reported problem is hyperactivity and urgency associated with bowel movements. Stools can be too loose and diarrhea-like if too much magnesium is taken. The solution is to reduce the amount that's supplemented.

As with other mineral supplements, a worsening in behavior or function may not be due to the element itself. It could be caused by the salt or mineral form, i.e., to the other chemical part(s) of the supplement. Magnesium citrate is notorious for causing loose stools and can be used therapeutically as a cathartic. Magnesium oxide that is not buffered may contain a bit of residual magnesium hydroxide, and upon dissolution, some ionized magnesium hydroxide could be formed. The result could be too alkaline (too high a pH for stomach acid to counter). Some residual magnesium hydroxide may be in other magnesium forms as well, including glycinate chelates. Magnesium that's taken with vitamins (at breakfast) usually has this acid-base pH problem dampened out by the other ingredients.

When the non-magnesium part of the supplement is suspected as causing trouble, the best thing to do is discontinue that kind or brand of supplement. Wait three or four days, then start with a different kind of magnesium. Form, amount and individual tolerance are all important to magnesium supplementation.

As with calcium, if oxalate excess persists while B_6, folic acid, taurine and lipase are being supplemented, then use of magnesium glycinate is not a good idea if other supplements bring the total glycine in supplements up to a gram or more.

About Magnesium (Optional Reading)

Magnesium is the activator of many enzymes in the body, particularly those needed for sugar and phosphate metabolism, and for energy transfer. Creatine and adenosine can't do energy delivery work without magnesium. This element also is essential for ionic balance in and around cells, and for assembly of substances that do antioxidant and detoxication work. Some magnesium-dependent enzymes have especially important jobs –

- To make SAM from methionine (enzyme: methionine adenosyltransferase). Methionine, when converted to SAM, becomes the big-time methyl donor in body tissues. It gives away a methyl to change the character of many molecules that are methyl acceptors. Examples are the methylation of (acetylated) serotonin to make melatonin, methylation of guanidinoacetate to make creatine, and methylation of lysine to start carnitine assembly.

- To make activated sulfur forms required for sulfation, a major detoxication process.
- To enable ATP to phosphorylate all the nucleosides, making them nucleotides: guanosine to GMP, GDP, GTP, cytidine to CMP, CDP, CTP, uridine to UMP, UDP, UTP, etc.
- To assemble glutathione from its three component amino acids: cysteine, glycine and glutamic acid.

Selenium, Se

Selenium is another trace element that's nutritionally essential. This one helps vitamin E do better with oxidants, and it is necessary for thyroid hormone formation – it activates the enzyme that forms T_3 from T_4. Selenium's antioxidant duty includes promotion of glutathione's action of neutralizing oxidizing agents.

Indications of Need

Quantitative elemental analyses of hair or blood cells usually are valid tests of Se status. A functional laboratory test for Se activity as an enzyme activator is measurement of glutathione peroxidase activity in red blood cells. Symptoms and conditions that are consistent with need for supplemental selenium are: chronic or frequent episodes of inflammation, past or current exposure to environmental substances expected to cause oxidant stress (toxicants), and occasionally, hypothyroidism. Usually, some problem other than low Se is at fault in hypothyroidism, and selenium deficiency is uncommon in the ASD population per my experience.

When and How Much

The supplemental form that I prefer is seleno-L-methionine. Most amino acid chelate forms also are active, and particularly beneficial is high-selenium yeast (a form of brewers' yeast). I'm less impressed by mineral selenates and selenites (including sodium forms).

Here are some supplemental guidelines for selenium from the Food and Nutrition Board of the USNRC.*

Age (years)	Micrograms/day
1-3	20 mcg/d
4-6	20 mcg/d
7-10	30 mcg/d
Males 11-14	40
Males 15-18	50
Females 11-14	45
Females 15-18	50

*10th Ed RDA, NRC, National Academy Press, 1989

As with iodine, I favor multivitamin/multimineral supplements with selenium included, in amounts not exceeding 100 micrograms/day. If you intend to supplement with stand-alone selenium in amounts exceeding 100 mcg/d, please confer first with your doctor or nutritionist about the advisability.

Adverse Responses to Selenium

Selenium toxicity has occurred with excessive supplementation and because of mistakes in labeling amounts. We're talking micrograms (mcg or µg), not milligrams (mg). Depending on chemical form, one milligram (1000 micrograms) used daily can cause selenium toxicity in an adult. Signs and symptoms of selenium excess include garlic-like breath, brittle nails, broken strands of hair, loss of hair, skin rash, fatigue, and irritability.

There are a few individuals who have sensitivity to selenium products with allergy-like symptoms. This is unusual. I've not heard of other adverse reactions to selenium as long as nutritionally correct amounts are used.

About Selenium (Optional Reading)

There are three important uses that our bodies have for selenium.
1. One function is activation of the enzyme glutathione peroxidase, which controls glutathione's ability to neutralize peroxides. Peroxides are oxidizing agents that, in excess, will damage tissue; they are made as a natural consequence of our metabolism and as a consequence of contamination by toxic or infectious agents. There is no getting away from peroxides in our tissues, so glutathione has to be active enough to limit the amount of peroxide – all the time. That means adequate selenium – all the time.

2. If you read the previous section on iodine, you learned that formation of the most active thyroid hormone, T_3, is made from thyroxine, T_4, by a selenium-containing enzyme. Thyroid function is absolutely selenium-dependent.

3. Selenium activates some enzymes in the antioxidant arsenal called "thioredoxin reductases". Thioredoxin is a big, body-made peptide; the name "thioredoxin" comes from what it is and does. It's "thio" because it contains sulfur, and it's "redoxin" because it's involved in chemical reduction and oxidation. Thioredoxins contain adjacent active sulfur-hydrogen parts (-SH, sulfhydryl) that can rescue and recycle oxidized proteins. When that happens, the thioredoxin peptide gets oxidized. The oxidation that occurs is direct joining of the two sulfur atoms following loss of their hydrogen atoms. In the oxidized form, thioredoxin can't rescue anything more. The enzyme that takes hydrogens from NADPH and puts them back on the sulfur to regenerate thioredoxin is thioredoxin reductase, and this enzyme contains and needs selenium to do its work. Sometimes, oxidized vitamin C is rescued (reduced) by thioredoxin reductase.

There's also the possibility that a selenium supplement can make a mercury contamination less toxic. Sometimes this is true, but it's a double-edged sword. According to published studies (experiments) with animals, Se can help to protect tissue from some severe toxic effects of inorganic mercury, such as renal tubular and intestinal necrosis, nephritis and some neurotoxicity. Mercury chloride is an inorganic form of mercury as opposed to methyl or ethyl mercury, which are organic forms for which there is no convincing evidence of Se protection. The less-toxic Se-Hg complex is stored in the liver and other organs, from which it is excreted at a very slow rate. Detoxification (chelation) therapy to remove mercury can be expected to go more slowly with Se-Hg than otherwise. The other edge of the sword is vastly increased selenium toxicity with the presence of inorganic mercury. If you use too much selenium, and have an inorganic mercury contamination, you get worse! Use of selenium to counter mercury contamination is a medical issue – please leave that use to your doctor. Frankly, I don't have a favorable opinion of selenium supplementation for this purpose.

Selenium is detoxified by methylation and SAM is the methyl source. By now, you know that's a problem for many with ASD. This is another reason to go easy and carefully with selenium supplementation.

Thirty years ago, I investigated the selenium-dependent enzyme, glutathione peroxidase, in autistics and found it to be subnormal; others also found this. My first response was to look for selenium deficiency. Except for a few individuals, I did not find such a deficiency in autistics by either hair or packed RBC analyses. Since then, various investigations by others have not produced convincing evidence that selenium is subnormal in autistics as a group. The hair element study by Adams, et al., discussed in the iodine section, found nearly identical hair selenium levels for the ASD group and the control group (each averaged). I believe that the occurrence of selenium deficiency in ASD is not noticeably different from the general population.

This leaves us with the curious dilemma of subnormal glutathione peroxidase activity for many with ASD. Selenocysteine is a newly discovered amino acid which has selenium in its chemical structure instead of sulfur, and a few proteins are assembled with selenocysteine instead of regular sulfur cysteine. Glutathione peroxidase, thyroid hormone deiodinase (T_4-to-T_3) and thioredoxin reductase are all selenocysteine proteins. Do some with autism have insufficient selenocysteine? I believe that some serious research needs to be done on this question. Mercury is documented to hinder glutathione peroxidase activity, so maybe part of the problem is mercury, at least in the past when thimerosal was in use.

When analyzing for selenium status, red blood cell assay is good, as is hair, except that hair is a lagging indicator. It reflects what was high, low or normal last month (using the inch next to the scalp for analysis). Blood serum, plasma and urine are not reliable indicators of selenium status.

Zinc, Zn

Zinc's primary role in the body is as an activator of enzymes. Several decades ago, some investigators believed that zinc deficiency was a major cause of autism. Such thinking comes from connecting theoretical dots to construct a theoretical picture of what's wrong. Zinc activates some peptidase digestive enzymes, and dietary peptides can be a problem in autism. This element is used by the enzyme that phosphorylates vitamin B_6 to make its active, coenzyme form, and many with autism benefit from supplemental B_6. Zinc activates methylation of homocysteine using trimethylglycine (TMG) to make methionine and DMG. An important adenosine processing enzyme requires zinc, and stabilization of RNA and DNA involves zinc. I could go on, listing dozens of metabolic processes that depend on zinc. Unfortunately for us, causes of autism and ASD aren't as simple as one deficient essential mineral. Subnormal zinc with subnormal zinc-enzyme function does occur in ASD and is an aggravating circumstance that we often have to deal with. But fixing zinc status is just one step along the journey to improvement.

Indications of Need

Most indicative is subnormal zinc as measured by blood cell or plasma analysis (against a correct reference range). Urine zinc is not indicative because 95% (approx) of zinc assimilated from the diet leaves via bile and fecal matter. Hair zinc is perverse as an indicator. Often, an elevated level of zinc in hair signifies maldistribution and poor utilization of the element. If you have a hair element test with high or low zinc, investigate further. The Adams et al. publication on hair element levels (Biol Trace Element Res. 2006) showed average zinc from ASD children at 11% higher than that of the control group average. While not statistically significant, I'd bet some of the ASD group had some maldistribution of zinc or deficient zinc function.

Signs or symptoms consistent with zinc deficiency: diminished acuity of taste and smell, poor appetite, pica, slow visual adaptation to darkness, growth retardation, skin rash, suppressed immune response, slow healing of wounds, and ataxia.

What Kind, When, and How Much?

The human mother's form of zinc (in breast milk) is zinc citrate – hard to beat that form. Other forms that I have had good experience with include: zinc-amino acid chelate (usually glycine), gluconate, alpha-ketoglutarate, and acetate which has very high bioavailability but is a prescription item. Zinc picolinate is a popular supplement form, but the picolinate part of the supplement may be a bit untrustworthy. There's some evidence that it abandons zinc before absorption and mates up with undesirables if they're in the neighborhood – lead, for instance. Zinc aspartate is questionable, too. Aspartate is somewhat like glutamate in its neuronal activities. Don't use zinc sulfate orally. That one hydrolyzes into a strong acid and base and may cause stomach upset.

For someone with ASD, zinc is best given away from meals. That's because there's some possible interference with the digestive enzyme dipeptidylpeptidase IV (DPP4), the enzyme that digests casomorphin peptides and other dietary peptides rich in proline. With reasonable amounts of zinc (15-30 mg/d), inhibition of DPP4 should be negligible. But with ASD, it's still good practice to give zinc away from food. Zinc is better absorbed that way, too. Evening is a good time for the zinc supplement, but don't give it when relatively large amounts of calcium are also given.

The low-dose starting level could be 5 mg/day for a small child, but most commercial supplements have 15 mg as the smallest unit dose or capsule content. 15 mg/day is the US FDA RDI (serving amount) for zinc.

The amounts of zinc that usually are safe and effective are tabulated below. Your doctor may wish to increase these amounts. Some individuals do require more, but I ask questions when children take more than 30 mg/d and adults take more than 60mg/d.

Weight		Zinc, mg/day
Kg	Lb	
20	44	5-15
30	66	7-20
40	88	10-30
50	110	12-35
60	132 and over	15-45

The Autism Research Institute has kept a tally of successes and failures with zinc supplement use in autism per parent responses (ARI Publication 34/March 2009):

Zinc Parent-Response Tally, responses = 2738		
Behavior or Traits Improved	No Discernible Effect	Behavior or Traits Worsened
54%	44%	2%

Sometimes it's very difficult to correct a zinc deficiency that's indicated by a blood or blood cell analysis. Supplements containing zinc, or stand-alone zinc supplements, just don't bring the level up to a satisfactory degree. What might help?

• Do give oral glutathione if it's tolerated. And a small dose of L-histidine can help too; histidine can complex and transport zinc. But it can do this for copper, too, so don't use histidine with food when the objective is both to lower copper and to raise zinc levels. Beneficial amounts would be 25 to 50 mg of glutathione (GSH) and 100 to 200 mg of L-histidine with 15 mg of zinc. WARNING: About one in 250 to 500 autistics has a metabolic condition known as histidinemia/histidinuria – too much histidine already. You'll only know this by doing an amino acid analysis. Do not give histidine when histidinemia is present. If you do try use of histidine with zinc, then give these between meals, midmorning or midafternoon. Histidine in the evening may cause insomnia.

- Watch for urinary zinc loss during detoxification treatments that use chelating agents. Some (D-penicillamine and EDTA) are known to remove zinc, and others may have that effect in an autistic individual whose sulfur and elemental biochemistries are abnormal. Larger supplemental doses of zinc may be needed at appropriate times during detoxification therapy.

- A physician may opt to use zinc acetate, a zinc form with very high bioavailability. It has FDA-approved orphan drug status for copper overload conditions. The pharmacy handbook, Facts and Comparisons should have the latest status of zinc acetate.

- Zinc often rises to satisfactory levels in blood serum or plasma before it does so in red blood cells. Much of erythrocyte zinc is bound to the cell membrane. If RBC zinc stays low, perhaps the cell membrane is deficient in certain fatty acids that should be present, or there's something wrong with membrane binding/transport of zinc. An RBC fatty acid analysis might be helpful. In cases like this, the supplemented amount of zinc is usually not the problem, it's insufficient binding to the cell membrane. It may be that toxicant chemicals, detoxication processes, or detoxification therapy is reducing zinc-membrane binding.

Adverse Response to Zinc?

It's hard to come up with a physiological reason for intolerance to zinc at low doses or dietary levels, or even to levels that are 2x or 3x the recommended amounts. One reason for problems would be copper deficiency, which is uncommon in the general or ASD population.

Copper and zinc compete for absorption, and extra zinc when copper levels are already marginal may cause a copper deficiency. Copper is needed for antioxidant protection (superoxide dismutase) and for dopamine and histamine metabolism. However, in my experience, subnormal copper findings by laboratory test are rare in autism/ASD. More likely, a worsening of behavior following a zinc supplement is due to the substance that the zinc is combined with. Trying a different form (such as switching from picolinate to gluconate or citrate) could solve the problem. Adverse reactions to large doses of zinc can occur, but such doses are well beyond what we have tabulated above.

About Zinc (Optional Reading)

Opinions about zinc status in autism have swung like a pendulum. Are you familiar with the expression "whale watching" when used to describe what's currently in vogue? Well, twice that I know of, zinc was an autism whale. Bernie Rimland once described to me how, in the 1960s, zinc deficiency was a major topic for parents of autistic children, and a few doctors, too, So much so, that some clinical studies were done. The findings of the first Defeat Autism Now! Conference in Dallas, Texas in January 1995 were recorded in a 1996 Consensus Report. That report includes mention of low zinc and of evidence of zinc dysfunction related to dietary peptide excesses. The low zinc findings were from clinical experience as reported by doctors who attended the conference. These opinions differ dramatically from conclusions published by Coleman and Gillberg in 1976. They reported <u>elevated</u> serum zinc in autistics versus controls. They found the autistic mean zinc concentration to be 171 mcg% (n=64), versus 112.5 mcg% for control individuals (n=69). In Coleman's studies, there was no statistically significant difference in serum copper concentrations: the population means were normal at about 120 mcg% for both autistics and controls.

A third go at the topic was carried out by Dr. William Walsh of the Pfeiffer Treatment Center in Illinois in about 2000. Walsh's findings disagreed with what was cited by Coleman and Gillberg and supported the previous but more anecdotal concept of relatively low zinc. Walsh reported in 2001 that the blood concentration ratio, serum copper ÷ plasma zinc was 1.63 for autistics (n=503) and 1.15 for age-matched controls (n=25)*. But, Walsh also stated that this relative copper/zinc excess was seen in 85% or 428 of the 503 subjects. Seventy five, or 15%, of the 503 did not have remarkably abnormal blood copper/zinc ratios. Not stated was how many of the 503 had absolutely low zinc per the laboratory reference range - Walsh WJ "Metallothionein in Autism" Pfeiffer Treatment Center, Naperville IL, (Oct 2001) as presented at the American Psychiatric Association Annual meeting, May 2001, New Orleans LA.

With the APA presentation by Walsh, zinc again became an autism "whale". Since then, interest in zinc and copper has waned considerably but it hasn't gone away. It's still a topic of concern. See also, Walsh, Usman and Tarpey, "Disordered Metal Metabolism in a Large Autism Population", *New Research Abstracts*, No. NR823, p 223, APA, May 2001.

These divergent findings, in my opinion, are due to several factors. First, the etiology of autism has changed from highly genetic with low incidence to highly environmental/acquired (including fetal and infant exposure) and high incidence. Numerically, it has grown from 3 to 6 per 10,000 births in the 1950s, to 90 to 100 per 10,000 births now). There are now many with ASD who also have intestinal disorder with inflammation and indications of brain inflammation as well. With inflammation, and especially with chronic infection (as may be present in the gut tissue with dysbiotic flora), copper is redistributed from the liver to the blood. A quantity known as leukocyte endogenous mediator may be involved, and its role in redistributing copper is a normal physiological response to infection and inflammation. This process increases blood copper levels and may even cause hypercupremia in acute infectious response. So, part of the remedy for lowering or normalizing blood copper/zinc ratio is to stop the inflammatory process.

What about findings of absolutely low zinc, as opposed to ratios? I've seen it often; it's real, not imaginary; but Zn deficiency is far from universal in ASD. One probable reason for zinc deficiency is the maldigestion/malabsorption that we see in some untreated cases. It does happen, but it's a shark, not a whale.

Literature – Minerals

National Research Council, <u>Recommended Dietary Allowances</u>, 10th Ed, National Academy Press, Wash DC 1989

Shils, Olsen and Shike, <u>Modern Nutrition in Health and Disease</u> Lea & Febiger, multiple editions – 1990s

Nielsen F "Ultratrace Elements in Nutrition" *Ann Rev Nutr* 4 (1984) 21-41

Ashmead A "The Metabolism of Amino Acid Chelates" Albion Laboratoris, Clearfield UT

Perchlorate articles (Iodine): *Chemical and Engineering News*:

May 5, 2003, p 11 "Of Lettuce and Rocket Fuel"

Aug 18, 2003, p 37 "Rocket-Fueled River

Jan 17, 2005, p 13 "Setting a Safe Dose for Perchlorate"

Sept 26, 2005 p 35 "Federal Policy on Perchlorate Evolves"

Feb 7, 2011 p 6 "Changing Course on Perchlorate – EPA will set drinking water standards for the rocket-fuel chemical"

~Introduction to Probiotics~

One goal of dietary intervention is reduction of the amount of incompletely digested food that can find its way to the lower small intestine and the large bowel. Such food promotes dysbiosis – growth of the wrong microorganisms in the intestines. Dysbiosis leads to infection, inflammation, increased permeability of intestinal mucosal tissue, and increased absorption/uptake of toxicants. Digestive enzyme use is a big help in achieving the goal of more complete digestion of food. But supplemented enzymes do not do the whole job of intestinal cleanup and maintenance of healthy flora.

Sometimes, the flora that's already in place can adapt to changes in food supply that might occur when diet is changed or when digestive enzyme supplements are used. Adapt usually means some dieoff while others change their lifestyle to cope with what's available. Adaptation can produce some quite aggressive and nasty microorganisms. An example is Candida yeast that morphs from a colony of oval clusters into a fungal infection featuring a network of threadlike tubes that try to invade the mucosal lining of the intestines. That type of invasive candida is hungry for a good meal and it will try to get it from you if it can't get it from your food. This happens with C. albicans after its easily-gotten food supply of glucose and cysteine are restricted. What is needed is another, friendly biotic organism that keeps these bad ones in check. We call these friendlies "probiotics". Besides defending against harmful flora, probiotic organisms help with immune defense and the supply of essential nutrients, and some change food substances into more useful forms. Some can make pantothenate and biotin, some make choline from lecithin, some digest complex sugars into simple ones (lactose or milk sugar into glucose and galactose), and some make natural antibiotic substances that work against growth of gut pathogens.

Indications of Need

- When you change the diet
- When you start to use digestive enzymes
- When a laboratory report on a stool analysis shows imbalanced or pathogenic flora
- When a stool analysis indicates maldigestion
- When a laboratory report on intestinal permeability shows excessive transfer of test substances into the blood ("leaky gut")

- When chemical markers consistent with intestinal dysbiosis are high in urine per a laboratory report (DHPPA, IAG, indoleacetic acid, phenylacetic acid, succinic acid, citramalaic acid, others)
- Chronic or frequent diarrhea
- Chronic or frequent constipation
- During any detoxification treatment
- While using antibacterial herbal supplements such as thyme or oregano
- During and after use of antibiotic medications.

When and How Much

The "when" is pretty much covered above (*Indications*) in terms of times of need. During daily activities, the best time to take a probiotic supplement is between meals and washed down with lots of water. That reduces loss of colony-forming units due to stomach acidity and digestion. Colony-forming units (CFU) are the live-count numbers that measure probiotic potency. I do not recommend use of enteric-coated probiotic supplements for those with ASD, because too often pancreatic function isn't sufficient to allow release of the organisms – more about this later. For most of the probiotic supplements that we're concerned with for ASD, we're talking billions of CFU. Examples (for 4 to 12 year olds) are –

Probiotic Organism	Daily serving, CFU
Lactobacillus rhamnosis	2 to 10 billion
Lactobacillus acidophilus	1 to 5 billion
Lactobacillus plantarum	1 to 5 billion
Bifidobacter bifidum	1 to 5 billion
Saccharomyces boulardii	0.5 to 3 billion

In all matters of how much, your doctor or nutritionist has the deciding vote. In my opinion, products containing less than the range of CFUs above are seldom helpful, except for young children. More than the CFU range may be beneficial in some cases, but need for really high CFU amounts (20 billion, 50 billion) means something is very wrong in the gastrointestinal tract. Whatever that may be, it's unlikely to be cured by wheelbarrow-load amounts of probiotics. Continued use of very high CFU amounts without investigating what's really wrong is poor practice. Some suggestions on what to look for in those who derive benefit from huge CFU probiotic supplements are –
- Is a bicarbonate supplement needed, 45-60 minutes after eating? (This would indicate pancreatic dysfunction with acidic pH in the intestines, which will continually kill most flora.)
- Was the probiotic that was initially used really at label potency? Is the one now being used really at label potency? Ask about this because, in my experience, many aren't. They may have been when manufactured but time, temperature and air (oxidation, moisture) all accelerate the death rate of these organisms. Under optimal storage conditions, a loss of 5% per month may occur.

• Check bowel transit time and diet. Probiotics can't stop rapid bowel transit when it's caused by food reactivity. Check for food allergy.

Adverse Responses to Probiotics

When first used, probiotic organisms may displace existing organisms, some of which are pathogenic or will become so when killed. The probiotic Streptomyces boulardii, for example, is especially adept at killing other yeasts. Lowering gut pathogenicity is good, but getting there often means worse before better. When pathogenic flora die off, their cells rupture and toxins are released. The same thing can happen when digestion is improved by dietary changes or by use of digestive aids (enzymes). Toxins from die-off can evoke symptoms, and one course of remedial action is oral use of activated charcoal, which absorbs the toxins and allows for their elimination in feces. **Activated charcoal** is best taken between meals and not at the same time as when nutritional supplements are given. One capsule of 250 mg charcoal between meals (midmorning and midafternoon) often does the job for young children. Over age 5 or 6 years, two, twice a day, may be needed. Putting charcoal on food to be eaten is a last-resort strategy. If necessary, stir it up in juice, to be taken between meals. Charcoal will darken the stools, sometimes turning them black. There's no harm in this. Do not use activated charcoal within an hour (before or after) of oral medications.

Symptoms to look for and that may be related to dieoff of dysbiotic flora include headache, which the child might not be able to tell you about, (increased) hyperactivity and stimming, diarrhea, general irritability and worsened sleep. While I mention these symptoms here, they may have already run their course when digestive enzymes were started or when a diet was tried., and you may not see any symptoms resulting from probiotic supplements.

I recommend that probiotic supplements be started gradually and ramped up in amount over a period of two weeks. The final target level is what your doctor or nutritionist advises or what the product label says. With most probiotics that I've had experience with, opening the gelatin capsule and sprinkling it on food to be immediately eaten works okay, but it's not as good as the between-meals-with-lots-of-water routine.

Other problems might arise from the stabilizing nutrients and additives in a particular brand of probiotics. If milk allergy is a problem, double check the dairy-free aspects of the brand you are using. Sometimes just changing the brand does the trick.

I do not recommend use of "enteric-coated" supplements for individuals with ASD, and this applies to probiotics. In order to work, enteric-coated supplements require normal or near-normal pancreatic function, which is what some with ASD don't have, especially early on in treatment. Among many other functions, the pancreas secretes bicarbonate into the upper small intestine where the partially-digested food (chyme) is acidic from stomach action. Enteric coatings are acid resistant and protect the capsule contents from acid attack – a good strategy for normal digestion. When the pH is raised from acidic to neutral or slightly alkaline (pH of 7 to 8) by bicarbonate, the pancreatic juices can dissolve the coating and the nutrients/probiotics are released. But this isn't happening for some with ASD, and probiotics that are enteric-coated don't get released.

About Selected Probiotic Organisms (Optional Reading)

There are many types of probiotic organisms, species, subspecies and "strains" that you will encounter if you explore the kinds that are sold. It is way beyond the scope of this book to describe the characteristics of all the probiotics organisms that are available. Instead, I will mention a select few and discuss some of the general characteristics that you should look for.

Probiotic organisms are sold in a dormant state with supporting nutrients included. The hope is that they will grow and multiply in the user's intestinal tract. Their implanting, growing and multiplying depend upon gut conditions. If pancreatic or biliary functions are poor and the pH conditions of the lower small intestine or large bowel are abnormal, there may be no growth or multiplication. If the diet is wrong, if there are too many active food allergies, if the pancreas doesn't put enough bicarbonate into the chyme, if bile synthesis is disordered, etc., then no brand of probiotics is likely to flourish. And virtually no live probiotics colonies can be cultured from the stool specimens of such individuals. This happens all too frequently with autistics, and hype about changing brands is just that – hype. In these cases you probably need a doctor's help to deal with food allergies, gastrointestinal dysfunctions, and to do laboratory tests that indicate the underlying problems.

Probiotic flora have a "shelf life" – they're dying off daily in the jar whether refrigerated or not. (Refrigeration helps considerably but doesn't stop this). Beware of brands that "don't require refrigeration". My experiences with these have been most disappointing. Such non-refrigerated types often exclude some of the most beneficial flora, such as Lactobacillus rhamnosis. Also, many of these have low counts of live CFUs when tested independently. So, keep the jar refrigerated and purchase a good brand (one that needs refrigeration) to start with.

Lactobacillus rhamnosis. This probiotic bacterium is very similar to "Lactobacillus GG" that is sold under the "Culturelle"™ brand name. Pure L. rhamnosis need not contain any casein or dairy products. L. rhamnosis was the "DDS#1" strain of Dr. Khem Shahani and the University of Nebraska Department of Dairy Science. For many years, rhamnosis was considered to be a dairy-free subtype of Lactobacillus acidophilus, and for a while after that it was thought to be "L. caseii". Given near-normal intestinal conditions, L. rhamnosis implants and colonizes vigorously in the mucosa of the lower part of the small intestine. Some claim that it colonizes in almost the entire small intestine. This would be an individual happenstance that depends on local conditions throughout the small intestine. L. rhamnosis does produce antibiotic-like substances which inhibit growth of some pathogenic flora, and that means rhamnosis acts synergistically with other probiotics. It grows on sugars such as rhamnose (which L. caseii does not), galactose, fructose, lactose, maltose and glucose. Rhamnosis is acid-resistant and most of it survives a pass through the stomach. It should be one of the first probiotics used after antibiotic therapy. Recent clinical research tells us that rhamnosis can also assist in getting rid of one of the pathological suspects in ASD – Clostridium difficile.

Lactobacillus acidophilus. Acidophilus is the "old reliable" in the world of probiotics. But if avoidance of dairy/casein is an objective, ask the vendor or manufacturer to certify that the product is dairy-free. Most L. acidophilus that's on the market is a dairy-based product that contains some casein. L. acidophilus produces acidophilin, a broad-spectrum antimicrobial that works against pathogens that might be in food. Like rhamnosis, acidophilus has been observed to decrease or stop diarrhea due to dysbiotic flora. Acidophilus can implant in the mucous membranes of the mouth, throat and small intestine. In women, it can grow in and protect the vaginal tract. Some strains require refrigeration; some do not. Regardless, refrigerating it will preserve its potency longer. Most strains are quite acid stable, and like rhamnosis, they survive normal stomach conditions.

Lactobacillus plantarum. Lactobacilli ferment milk and make lactate (lactic acid); they were discovered and categorized on the basis of which sugars they could live on and process into lactate. Plantarum is unusual in that it likes carbohydrates and sugars in cereal grains, rye especially, sourdough, also olives, pickles and several oriental vegetables. It produces an antibiotic, lactolin, and it is a big-time enemy of Candida albicans. Originally speciated and studied in the 1930s, this microorganism has attracted recent attention because it survives exposure to some medical antibiotics (tetracyclines), survives stomach acidity, and goes to work knocking out gas-producing intestinal bacteria including clostridia. As an added bonus, it reduces nitrates – a food-source oxidant. Ten years ago, few probiotic supplements contained any L. plantarum. We now know that its ability to modulate intestinal flora helps normalize motility and reduce irritability and inflammation in intestinal tissues. I strongly recommend inclusion of L. plantarum in probiotic supplements for ASD.

Bifidobacter bifidum. Bifidus, also called Bifidobacter lactis, is thought to produce a natural antibiotic similar to acidophilin, but bifidus colonizes in the large bowel below where acidophilus grows. So L. acidophilus and B. bifidum complement each other with respect to location and antimicrobial functions. Bifidobacterium anaerobes have been found to predominate in the colon of healthy breast-fed infants. Those who are not breast-fed may have little or no bifidobacteria to help with acid-base balance in the bowel. While bacterial action and putrefaction can produce ammonia, which is alkaline (high pH), B. bifidum reduces putrefaction and produces short-chain organic acids (acetic, lactic) which lower or normalize the pH. B. bifidum can be grown dairy-free and that may be the strain you require. Ask and be sure. Refrigeration may or may not be required for this one; refer to the product label. But again, refrigerating can help extend shelf life whether specified or not.

Saccharomyces boulardii. This is our "hired gun". It's a yeast, not a bacterium, and it kills other yeast such as Candida. S. boulardii is a subspecie type of Saccharomyces cerevisiae, which you may run across in reading about probiotics. The whole specie group are yeast killers. I do not recommend continual daily use of billion-plus CFU amounts. Effective, as-needed amounts of S. boulardii depend on the individual and whether potential yeast-fostering nutrients or supplements are also being used and how much. Yeast-fostering substances include alpha-lipoic acid, DMSA, cystine, cysteine and N-acetylcysteine, and sometimes glutathione.

Recently, S. boulardii has been reported to help eliminate intestinal Clostridium difficile, when used with other agents (special antibiotics, L. rhamnosis, L. plantarum). Sometimes S. boulardii is needed for two to three weeks a 2 billion CFU/day, sometimes twice that amount. The end point of need is when urine IAG, DHPPA and other pertinent urinary dysbiosis markers return to normal levels by lab test. Do not stop use prematurely just because symptoms of bowel irritability subside.

Boulardii does not colonize well in human intestine, and it dies out as its food supply diminishes. It is itself killed by antifungal medications Diflucan and Sporinox. S. boulardii probiotic formulations must be refrigerated to maintain potency. When blended with other probiotics (e.g. plantarum), there is minor but continual loss of the other probiotics. Usually, a responsible manufacturer will put an overage of other probiotics in with S. boulardii so that label CFU claims are met for at least six months. Out of date probiotic formulations with S. bouldardii should be discarded.

Literature - Probiotics

Friend BA and Shahani KM "Nutritional and therapeutic aspects of lactobacilli" *J. Appl Nutrition* 26 no.2 (1984) 125-153.

Marteau P, Pochart P et al. "Effect of chronic ingestion of a fermented dairy product containing Lactobacillus acidophilus and Bifidobacterium bifidum on metabolic activities of the colonic flora in humans" *Am.J.Clin Nutrition* 52 (1990) 685-688

Berg R, Bernasconi P et al. "Inhibition of Candida albicans translocation from the gastrointestinal tract of mice by oral administration of Saccaromyces boulardii" *J. Infect Dis* 168 no.5 (1993) 1315-1318

Salminen S, Isolauri E and Salminen E "Clinical uses of probiotics for stabilizing the gut mucosal barrier: successful strains and future challenges" *A van Leeuw J Microb* (Kluwer) 70 (1996) 347-358

Majumaa H and Isolauri E "Probiotics: a novel approach in the management of food allergy" *J.Allergy Clin Immunol* 99 no.2 (1997) 179-185

Wynne AG, McCartney AL et al. "An in vitro assessment of the effects of broad-spectrum antibiotics on the human gut microflora and concomitant isolation of a Lactobacillus plantarum with anti-Candida activities" *Anaerobe* 2004 Jun;10(3):165-9

Bixquert JM "Treatment of irritable bowel syndrome with probiotics" *Rev Esp Enferm Dig* 2009 Aug 101(8):553-64 (See PMID 19785495, Pub Med)

Taurine

Taurine is a conditionally-essential, amino acid-like nutrient with many important functions ranging from assisting brain development and neurotransmitter regulation to digestion and antioxidant duty. Don't ignore this one – it's really important and likely to be helpful. That's why it is suggested as a Tier 1 supplement.

Indications of Need

Poor sleep, persistent signs of oxidant stress or inflammation, seizures, clay-colored stools, reactivity to swimming-pool water, diagnosis of: elevated blood ammonia, excess stool fat, elevated oxalates (blood or urine), inadequacy of vitamin A or D or E or of essential fatty acids or cholesterol; magnesium deficiency, vitamin B_6 deficiency.

Abnormal levels of taurine measured by amino acid analysis in blood or urine always are suspicious. High taurine in blood plasma may be due to inflammation and cell damage while low often means that internal synthesis plus dietary supply are insufficient. High in urine is almost always due to urinary wasting. This can occur when there is intestinal bacterial dysbiosis (produces beta-alanine, which blocks renal conservation of taurine), excessive dietary intake of beta-alanine peptides (anserine, carnosine), or disorder with pyrimidine metabolism (possibly pervasive developmental disorder, "PDD"). In ASD, circumstantial evidence indicates that taurine can be high where it is measured but not needed (urine, for example) but low where it is needed but isn't measured (neutrophils, neurons, and brain tissue).

When and How Much?

Early on, often at the beginning of nutritional intervention, is a good time for you to try a taurine supplement. It seems to work especially well with breakfast in moderate amounts: 100 to 250 mg/d for 2 to 5 year olds and 250 to 500 mg/day for 6 to 12 year olds. Teens and adults may benefit from 500 to 1000 mg/d. I do not suggest daily supplements of taurine above 2000 mg for anyone.

Adverse Response to Taurine?

In my experience, adverse responses to appropriate amounts of taurine are very uncommon. During the more than 25 years that I have suggested taurine use, reports to me of problems have numbered less than a dozen (out of thousands who have tried taurine as a nutritional supplement). If the electrolyte levels are already imbalanced in a certain way and are not corrected by homeostasis, then taurine, in significant amounts, could worsen the imbalance. Intolerance can occur in hyperkalemia conditions (excessive blood potassium), Addison's disease, and insulin deficiency if gram quantities of taurine are used continuously. This is because taurine mediates the flux of electrolyte minerals across cell membranes. As with all supplements, start at a low level (100 or 250 mg/d depending on body weight or age). We are cautioned by clinical researchers not to use more than about 2000 mg/d (2 grams/day) and large amounts can produce effects that are opposite to what would be expected or hoped for. Once again, when used appropriately, reactivity or intolerance to taurine is rare.

About Taurine (Optional Reading)

On average, I found taurine to be deficient when I surveyed amino acid analyses of 32 autistic individuals in the early 1980s. I presented that finding (and low cysteine too) at the 1984 NSAC Annual Meeting. (NSAC is now the Autism Society, formerly ASA.) My study is published in the Proceedings of that meeting. Numerous clinicians have found it to be low compared with lab norms when reviewing amino acid analyses for their autistic patients. Recently taurine has again been measured to be low (in blood plasma) in a comprehensive nutritional analysis of autistic children versus a control population; in a study headed by Prof. James Adams of Arizona State University. (See Literature-Taurine for citation.) When I presented my findings of low taurine (1984), Sidney M. Baker, MD, presented a companion paper about how taurine supplementation benefited an autistic child in many ways, especially sleep. His clinical experience and case report also are recorded in the 1984 NSAC Meeting Proceedings.

In 1827, two Austrian scientists, Leopold Gmelin and Fredrich Tiedemann, published research that isolated and identified taurine in ox bile. Gmelin took the word "taurine" from the Latin name for ox, Bos taurus. Today, we are still learning about this remarkable "amino acid" which differs quite a bit from the 20 or so amino acids that link together to form proteins. Taurine's acid part is based on sulfur, not carbon, and while taurine can link with some other biochemicals to form peptide-like compounds, it is not included in proteins. It does, however, get measured along with regular amino acids in blood plasma or urine by laboratory amino acid analyses.

As a nutrient, taurine is conditionally essential for young children, which means that the internal process that makes it is immature and usually insufficient during the first few years of life. For the developing fetus and for neonates, internal formation doesn't begin to meet the demands, and taurine then is a strictly essential nutrient. It has to come from Mom via cord blood or milk, or from infant formula. What makes the stuff so essential? Here are some of the actions of taurine in our cells and organs along with some clinical and nutritional observations.

Uptake of Essential Lipids (Fats) In liver tissue, taurine combines with cholesterol to make an important part of bile – "taurocholate". Taurocholate and other bile components (including the glycine analog, glycocholate) facilitate the uptake of essential fats, fatty acids and glycerols from the small intestine. For most of our lives, adequacy of vitamins A,D,E and cholesterol is to some extent dependent on taurocholate. During infancy, uptake of these essential nutrients is very dependent on taurocholate. And while vitamin D is mostly made internally (from cholesterol), vitamin D also is conditionally essential, especially when sunlight is scarce, as in winter at latitudes beyond about 35° N or S, or when indoor activities prevail in lifestyle. Parents, if you have been advised to give vitamin D or cholesterol to your child, then I suggest that a little taurine be given as well.

An additional, potential problem with decreased uptake of dietary fat is increased uptake of oxalate from the diet. Some years ago, an independent researcher, Susan Owens, brought oxalate to our attention. Oxalate can be a dead-end product of amino acid (glycine) metabolism, and excessive amounts can be formed internally when certain metabolic imbalances occur. Oxalate also comes directly from the diet; high oxalate foods include spinach, chard, rhubarb, cocoa, green and wax beans, beets, sweet potatoes, cashews and almonds, figs, and most berries. One problem with oxalate is that, once inside the body, it combines with calcium to form an insoluble compound, a "stone". What's supposed to happen to most dietary oxalate is that it meets up with calcium in the intestine and forms calcium oxalate there. That oxalate doesn't get absorbed; it leaves the body with the fecal matter. This is where taurine becomes important. Taurine helps the transfer of dietary fat out of the intestines and into the body. If there's too much fat in the intestines, that fat binds the calcium, and then, oxalate is free to enter the bloodstream.

When I looked up "hyperoxaluria" (too much oxalate in urine) in *Harrison's Principles of Internal Medicine*, I found fat malabsorption reported as a major cause of excess oxalate uptake. Please refer to the lipase section of the Digestive Enzymes chapter for more information.

Glutamate-GABA Balance, Sleep, Seizures, Ammonia. Another important function of taurine is regulation of the balance between glutamic acid (glutamate) and gamma-aminobutyric acid (GABA). One neurotransmitter theory of autism is that glutamate neurotransmitter and/or receptor activity is excessive. High glutamate also is considered to be a cause of some types of seizures. Glutamate is a stimulatory neurotransmitter while GABA is inhibitory, or down-regulating for neuronal excitability. When glutamate activity is excessive, taurine is believed to counter this by promoting formation of glutamine from some of the glutamate. This brings glutamate more into balance with GABA. Several researchers have reported reduction of glutamate levels and some degree of improvement in certain seizure conditions following administration of taurine. The pioneering work of Dr. N van Gelder is an outstanding example. Online, PubMed now lists over 200 titles of publications linking taurine and seizures, some reporting remission, others not.

Potentially, there are several known reasons for poor sleep patterns in autism. Some important ones are inadequate melatonin and dysregulated adenosine metabolism. But when Dr. Sidney Baker used taurine to correct rapid transitioning of awake-sleep-awake-sleep-awake…. in a 15 year old boy (after he and others tried just about everything else in four prior years), I started to pay even more attention to it. I have to believe it was the glutamate-to-glutamine function of taurine, bringing down the stimulatory neurotransmitter glutamic acid that did the trick. Dr. Baker's case report on this can be found in the 1984 NSAC Annual Meeting Proceedings, pages 16-17.

What about seizures? Are they overemphasized in autism? I don't think so. At a recent DAN! meeting, Dr. Susan Swedo of NIMH reported EEG finding which showed that 30% to 60% of children/adolescents with autism have epilepsy to some degree. Most often, this has been identified by overnight EEGs that pick up various diffuse or multifocal or focal episodes that are not present or noticed while the individual is awake. (October 2008 Defeat Autism Now Conference, San Diego, see Conf. Proceedings, Science Session, pages 11-18, esp. page 17).

If an autistic person has seizures, watch out for high taurine in blood plasma. In my opinion, the high taurine could reflect a corrective compensation mechanism. In the textbook *Taurine* (Raven Press, 1976, editors Huxtable and Barbeau, page 297), Dr. van Gelder reports lowering glutamate levels by giving taurine to seizure patients when plasma taurine was already high. Dr. van Gelder found that giving taurine – irrespective of its initial or final blood plasma levels – restored the plasma levels of glutamic acid to normal.

Why is elevated blood ammonia an indication for taurine use? In the brain and CNS, ammonia is naturally detoxified by first combining it with alpha-ketoglutaric acid to make glutamic acid (glutamate). Glutamic acid then adds another ammonia (as an "amide") to form glutamine. Glutamine readily exits by crossing the brain-blood barrier, a transit that glutamic acid does too slowly. Taurine's role is to enhance the glutamic acid $\rightarrow$ glutamine transformation. Without this series of transformations, ammonia would accumulate, attack cell membranes, cause swelling ventricles and migraine. Ammonia intoxication can also cause slurred speech, disorientation, irritability; chronic elevations can lower IQ. Acute elevations of ammonia can be fatal. If your child has a diagnosis of elevated ammonia, keep the doctor in charge, don't try to treat this yourself.

Cell electrolyte balance and stabilization of cell membranes. Cells in our bodies are constantly passing electrolyte ions in and out as part of their efforts to maintain organ and tissue activity and health. Electrolyte elements are potassium, magnesium, sodium and calcium, and the ions are positively charged atoms of each. A positively-charged ion may be thought of as an atom that has lost one or more electrons. Chemists denote these as K^+, Mg^{++}, Na^+ and Ca^{++}. They are electrically balanced in our tissues by various negative ions such as chloride Cl^-, sulfate SO_2^{--} and bicarbonate HCO_3^-. Cell membranes contain chemical pumps and passageways ("channels") that operate ionic transfer processes.

When a neuron does its work in the brain, it takes in energy (fuel) as glucose but loses some calcium ions in the process. If the calcium isn't replaced, the depletion will soon prevent the neuron from operating. In the 1970s, Dr Welty and others at the U. of South Dakota, Dept. of Physiology and Pharmacology, reported on animal tissue studies which demonstrated that taurine modulated or controlled part of the ion transfer process. From their studies we know that taurine works to reverse the calcium-depleting effects of glucose in brain and heart cells, and to reverse potassium loss in heart tissues. Other studies by other investigators attribute similar, whole-body electrolyte balance to taurine. Adequate taurine in the kidneys provides a magnesium-sparing effect for the body.

Cellular Antioxidant. Inside some cells, such as white blood cells (neutrophils) taurine provides a crucial antioxidant function. These cells are defense cells for the body, and immunologists and cytologists call them phagocytes. They respond to alien stuff by trying to puncture, penetrate, envelop, digest, oxidize, etc. And what gets phagocytic cells going are any of the following –

- Bacteria (staph, strep, salmonella, enterobacter, proteus, klebsiella, microbacteria, others)
- Yeasts (candida, aspergillus)
- Wheat germ agglutinin, substances that "clump" cells
- Fine particles, organic & inorganic, engine & power plant exhausts
- Fluorides
- Some viruses (naked virus forms without lipid envelopes – rhinoviruses, papilloma, rotaviruses)

The oxidation part of cellular defense leads to generation of hypochlorous acid and the hypochlorite ion (OCl⁻), the same ion that's the active agent in household bleach. Hypochlorite will oxidize (inactivate or kill) just about anything. This includes the cell membrane and the cell itself if excesses of it aren't mopped up. Who's the mop? Yes, it's taurine. Taurine collects excess OCl⁻ by forming a stable, inert "chloroamine". Helping to cope with the oxidant action of neutrophils are vitamins C and E; they neutralize oxygen radicals (extremely reactive forms of oxygen with an unpaired electron and that typically find a reaction target in less than one ten thousandth of a second). This means that some taurine and vitamins C and E have to be in place in the phagocyte cell when it decides to attack some alien substance. There's no time for preparation; they have to be there on the spot.

Taurine is the most abundant, free-form amino acid in neutrophils of the "polymorphonuclear leukocyte" form (a type of phagocyte). Its concentration inside those cells normally is 10x more than the next most abundant amino acid (aspartic) - Bremer et al. *Disturbances of Amino Acid Metabolism: Clinical Chemistry and Diagnosis* 1981, p. 225 Table B24.

Taurine also is the most abundant free-form amino acid in a type of neurological cell – the astrocyte. Its role there isn't well understood as yet, but it's believed that neurons and astrocytes interact cooperatively to make taurine when it's needed.

Detoxication. Your body has cleanup processes called *detoxication* and your clinician has treatments called *detoxification*. Taurine has several major roles in detoxication. First, it combines with cholesterol to form taurocholate. That's part of bile (discussed above). Overall, taurine helps the body's cholesterol balance. It does so by helping dietary cholesterol get in, and by using some of it up. About half of cholesterol is eliminated from the body via fecal excretion after being converted to the bile salts taurocholate and glycocholate.

The biliary pathway itself is a major detoxication route for the body. Most oil- (lipid-) soluble wastes go out in bile, as do some toxicants of interest in autism. Much of glutathione-bound mercury and sulfated wastes (steroids, catechols, phenols, phenolics) are excreted that way, as are lead, arsenic, and metabolized forms of organochlorine and organophosphate pesticides and herbicides.

Finally, taurine combines with ("conjugates") some used-up or degraded lipid molecules, and one of particular interest is vitamin A, retinol. Degraded vitamin A is conjugated with taurine to form retinotaurine, which is expelled via bile and fecal matter. Some years ago, megadose vitamin A was proposed as a beneficial nutrient for autism, one reason being that it is an anti-infective agent that might protect against or lessen the effects of viral infection. If you are concerned about vitamin A dosage, one precaution is to supplement taurine.

Regulator of Neurological Development. As a regulator of cellular electrolytes, and probably because of other yet-to-be-described functions, taurine is believed to influence development of the brain and nervous system during fetal and neonatal periods. More about this follows.

Taurine in Fetus and Neonate (Optional Reading)

Doctors John Sturman and Gerald Gaull of Mt. Sinai School of Medicine, New York City, wrote a wonderful review of taurine in the developing brains of humans (and Rhesus monkeys) in the book <u>Taurine</u>, previously referenced. Here are some of the highlights.

When the human fetus is small, occipital lobe taurine concentration is 5 to 7 micromoles per gram of occipital tissue. This is thought to be 500 to 700% higher than for adult humans. As the fetus' brain grows, the taurine concentration decreases continually, but remains significantly higher than adult human levels. Shortly after birth (days), the occipital lobe taurine level has been measured to be only about 1 micromole per gram. Liver tissue studies show a very similar pattern with taurine concentration in liver tissue dropping from 3 to 5 micromoles per gram during gestation to 1 micromole/gram four days after birth. What's happening here?

My review of the literature on this leads to the conclusion that fetal taurine comes mostly from mom, and she both makes it and gets it in her diet. Taurine is in meat, fish and fowl; it's quite abundant in shellfish. Taurine can be made enzymatically from cysteine or cystine. These amino acids can also be of dietary origin or can be formed via a sequence of chemical changes to the essential amino acid methionine.

Making taurine from cysteine requires a chemical transformation controlled by an enzyme with a long name: cysteine sulfinic acid decarboxylase, or "CSAD" for short.

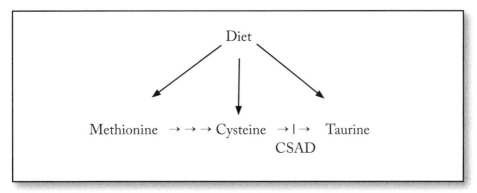

CSAD is the rate-limiting enzyme for taurine formation, and it has little if any activity in the fetus. During early infancy, its activity increases, but it still isn't high enough to provide all the taurine that's needed. Hence, in infancy taurine is conditionally essential. By the way, CSAD requires coenzyme pyridoxal 5'-phosphate (from vitamin B_6) to do its enzyme work. That's why a diagnosis or a suspicion of vitamin B$_6$ need can also be an indication of taurine need.

After birth, of course, the transfer system for taurine, mom-to-fetus, is gone. It was particularly active in the three to four weeks prior to birth when the fetus accumulated 6 to 8 milligrams of taurine per day. So, what happens after birth? Well, it's mom to the rescue again – with breast milk. Human breast milk is very rich in taurine. Cows' milk from the store is not.

Premature-birth neonates lack the reserve of taurine that normally accumulates in the weeks just before birth, so preemies may benefit from extra taurine. In Germany, two clinical researchers, Drs. Berger and Gobal, studied exactly this (*Monatsschr Kinderheilkd.* 140 (1992) 416-421, article in German). In a study of 22 preemies born during the 30th -35th week of gestation and requiring parenteral feeding, Berger and Gobal found that a 50 mg/kg body wt. per day supplement was required to match the blood taurine level of breast-fed neonates.

Now that you've learned about cysteine sulfinic acid decarboxylase (CSAD), I can say a little more about taurine's role in neuronal communication where it's made to meet demand – like burgers at a fast-food restaurant. In our brains, the tiny electrical charge that's essential for neuronal activity opens a channel that lets calcium ions leave the cell (neuron); a normal happening in neuronal electrochemistry. The calcium ions act on an enzymatic process (phosphorylation) to activate CSAD and make taurine. And taurine aids replenishment of neuronal calcium. By feedback regulation, when taurine accumulates, it shuts down CSAD. Taurine then is dispersed or metabolized so that it won't inhibit CSAD during the next round of neuronal activity. However, if for some reason brain CSAD can't make taurine, then it seems to me that neuronal communication – and neuronal network development - will be in trouble. If you have a research interest in the dynamics of taurine formation in the brain, there's a research publication on this: Wu J-Y, W Chen et al. "Mode of Action of Taurine and Regulation Dynamics of its Synthesis in the CNS" *Advances in Experimental Medicine and Biology* book series, 483 (Taurine 4) Springer (Netherlands) 2002 35-44.

As mentioned earlier, bile taurocholate and glycocholate (from glycine) are needed to have adequate uptake of dietary lipids such as cholesterol, vitamin A, and essential fatty acids. But for the breast-fed infant, taurocholate has to do the whole job! Only after weaning does glycine as glycocholate begin to take over some of this function. What about cows' milk? Well, right after a calf is born, a cow's milk is rich in taurine, too. But we humans don't get that milk; the calf does. After prolonged lactation, and after the calf is weaned, the taurine content of cows' milk has declined significantly and is only about 10% of what human mom makes for her newborn.

Did we always understand this? No. Not until 1984 was taurine added to infant formula following the revelation that it is an essential nutrient for human infants – essential for development of retinal, brain, and liver tissues.

Food Sources of Taurine

Food	Milligrams of Taurine per four (4) ounces of food**
Clams*	275
Oysters*	80
Tuna*	75
Pork	60
Lamb	55
Beef	40
Chicken	40
Human milk	60
Cow's milk	7

* Beware of mercury content
** Taurine amount can vary +/- 20%

Adapted from Hayes KC and EA Trautwein, "Taurine", Chapt. 31 in Shils, Olson and Shike, Eds. Modern Nutrition in Health and Disease, Lea & Febiger Pub., 1994.

Taurine in the Infant and Young Child, What Can Go Wrong

Aside from dietary inadequacy and CSAD immaturity, what can go wrong with taurine supply? Actually, quite a lot. Here's some of it.

Persistent inflammation and oxidant stress can result in cysteine being detoured away from taurine formation and toward glutathione synthesis. Changes in gene expression in response to inflammation (epigenetic changes) can throttle down cysteine sulfinate levels such that CSAD might have little material to work with. If glutathione function is disordered, as it appears to be for many with autism, and if the biochemical messengers for oxidant stress (cytokines) are continually elevated, the resulting maladaptive state could feature chronic taurine inadequacy. Maldigestion, malabsorption, food intolerances and intestinal dysbiosis can contribute to inflammation and to limited formation of taurine. In contrast, special diets, supplemental digestive enzymes, and anti-inflammatory strategies can be helpful to taurine formation.

Toxicant damage to enzymes or transport mechanisms _combined with genetic variance_ can limit internal formation of taurine. For autism, there now are numerous measured, inferred, and hypothesized disorders in the metabolic sequence that makes taurine: methionine → → →cysteine → → taurine. The possible disorders involve inhibited transport mechanisms, inadequate vitamin cofactors, genetic variants and epigenetics (changes to gene expression caused by acquired stressors) and toxicants including organophosphates (pesticides, nerve agents), mercury, lead and antimony.

Elevations of an unusual amino acid, beta-alanine, can result in urinary loss of taurine. Taurine and beta alanine look similar to kidney tubules, and excessive taurine winds up in the urine when beta-alanine is elevated in blood or urine. I've often observed elevated urine taurine in autistic individuals along with elevated beta-alanine. While urine (and blood) taurine levels may be normal or abnormal, it's important to realize that cellular and organ levels are really what matter most. Unfortunately we can't measure those levels with conventional laboratory tests.

What causes elevated beta-alanine? (a) Excessive dietary intake of anserine and carnosine peptides (chicken, turkey, duck, tuna, salmon, beef, pork); (b) Bacterial infection or dysbiosis ; (c) Pyrimidine metabolism disorder with accelerated metabolic formation of beta-alanine. Pyrimidine metabolism disorder is reported to underlie some types of Pervasive Developmental Disorder" (PDD).

To confound the issue of taurine adequacy, elevated blood levels also occur. Generally, blood cell levels of taurine are much higher than blood plasma levels. But if cell breakage is occurring or if tissue inflammation is present, plasma can gain taurine from injured cells. Also, if glutamic acid (glutamate) goes up, one defense mechanism is to have taurine go up, too. The bottom line on taurine levels in blood plasma and/or urine is to be wary of high or low readings. Both situations can indicate functional insufficiency of taurine in the cell environments where it matters most.

If vitamin B$_6$ as pyridoxal 5'-phosphate is truly deficient, then CSAD can't do its part to make taurine.

Cystinuria, an inherited disorder in renal processing of cystine resulting in urinary wasting of cystine, might limit taurine formation. However, dietary taurine (from mom) may compensate in infancy, and regular food sources may compensate later in life. Of the thousands of amino acid analyses on ASD children that I've reviewed, I can only remember two or three with signs of cystinuria – so I mention this only for completeness. The condition may only be a coincidence, with an incidence like that of the general population.

During brain development, some toxicants might cause disordered neuronal electrolyte levels and interfere with neuronal action, synchrony and architecture, regardless of taurine levels. According to Casarett & Doull's <u>Toxicology</u> text, some organochlorines and pyrethroids act as neurotoxins and are documented to disorder neuronal electrolyte, energy, and polarization processes. Example environmental toxicants of this type are (or have been) DDT, dicofol, endosulfan and dieldrin.

Literature – Taurine

Huxtable R and A Barbeau eds, <u>Taurine</u> Raven Press, NY, 1976

<u>PDR for Nutritional Supplements</u>, Thompson/PDR 2001, Thompson PDR, Montvale NJ p 442-445

Hayes K and E Trautwein, "Taurine" Chapt. 31 in Shils, Olson and Shike, eds, <u>Modern Nutrition in Health and Disease</u>, 8th ed, Lea & Febiger, NY 1994

Scriver C and T Perry "Disorders of Omega-Amino Acids in Free and Peptide Forms" Chapt. 26 in Scriver et al. eds. <u>The Metabolic Basis of Inherited Disease</u> 6th Ed. McGraw-Hill (1985) 755-760

Pangborn JB, Proceedings 1984 NSAC (now ASA) Annual Conference, San Antonio TX, 32-51. (Taurine/cysteine discussion pages 44-46).

Adams JB et al. "Nutritional and Metabolic Status of Children with Autism vs Neurotypical Children, and the Association with Autism Severity" *Nutrition and Metabolism* 2011, 8:34

Forehand J et al. "Inherited Disorders of Phagocyte Killing" Chapt 114 in Scriver et al. eds, op.cit.

Bremer H et al. <u>Disturbances of Amino Acid Metabolism: Clinical Chemistry and Diagnosis</u>, Urban and Schwarzenberg, Munich 1981, articles on taurine

~Introduction to Vitamins~

The word vitamin is a contraction of "vital amine", a phrase used a century ago to recognize and categorize a group of dietary nutrients that are essential for health and life. "Amine" refers to the nitrogen content of the earliest-found members of this nutrient group. When first used, the name "vitamine" was applied to vitamin B_1 (thiamine) by Casimer Funk, who isolated it in 1911. But to keep the record straight, Funk wasn't first to identify B_1. Umetaro Suzuki did that in 1910, following up on the 1884 observation of Admiral Takaki (Surgeon General of the Japanese Navy) that some of his sailors got beriberi on extended voyages, and that the disease was relieved by a complete diet – something essential was missing from a sailor's diet at sea, and some years later Dr. Suzuki went looking for it.

Today, "vitamin" refers to a broader class of essential nutrients. Some, the B-vitamins, contain nitrogen and are amines. Vitamins A, C, D and E do not contain nitrogen. Vitamins make things happen, but they are not extensively involved in the body's structure, which distinguishes them from other vital amines, the essential amino acids.

Another distinction is this: if animals are fed only pure proteins, fats, carbohydrates, and essential minerals, they don't live very long. Vitamins are the additional nutrients needed for health and life.

B-vitamins act as enzyme helpers. Enzymes are proteins that are catalysts for chemical change in our cells, organs and tissues. They promote transformations among the substances that allow our bodies to grow, function, repair and rebuild as necessary for good health.

Not all enzymes require vitamin helpers. When they do, the nutrient form of the vitamin must undergo chemical changes to become a helper or "coenzyme". Coenzymes attach to pre-enzyme proteins (apoenzymes) to form complete or whole enzymes (holoenzymes). Only then does the combination have the catalytic ability that's required to promote the transformations our bodies need. The substances that the enzymes act on are called reactants or substrates, and the transformed materials are the products of the enzymatic process.

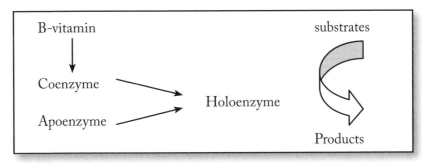

The vast majority of enzymatic processes in the human body do not require coenzymes – but many important ones do. Typically, the body is unable to synthesize vitamins or

coenzymes without dietary input of starting nutrients. Two exceptions are vitamin D and coenzyme forms of vitamin B_3, "niacin". Niacin forms can be made in limited amounts from the nutritionally essential amino acid tryptophan, and vitamin D can be made from cholesterol, but sunlight is required along the way. Because we don't make enough of these essential substances, they are required in the diet to some extent and are considered to be vitamins as well.

There are many vitamin functions besides the coenzyme actions of B-vitamins. Vitamin A influences cell differentiation (what cells become when they mature), helps immune response, works to maintain membrane integrity, including keeping skin healthy, and participates in the chemistry of vision. Vitamin C acts as an antioxidant. It enhances chemical transformations involving hydrogen bound to oxygen (hydroxylation) such as with formation of carnitine, collagen tissue and metabolism of dopamine. Vitamin D has hormonal functions that regulate calcium metabolism and gene transcription functions. Vitamin E has antioxidant and membrane protection functions different from those of vitamins C and A. In general, vitamins are team players. They are efficient at assisting one another in maintaining health, but they are usually unable to substitute for each other.

Vitamins and Autism

Is autism caused by a vitamin deficiency? In my opinion, no; that generality goes way too far. Can some autistics benefit in functional and behavioral ways from vitamin supplements? Yes, many definitely can.

Since Chris and I were informed of the diagnosis of autism for our son (1970), I've watched intently as hypotheses about autism and vitamins have hopscotched from one to another. Vitamin B_6, vitamin C, folate, folate with B_{12}, vitamin A, B_{12} without folate, vitamin B_1, B_{12} as methylcobalamin, and recently vitamin D have all had their turn in the spotlight. Each time, rather exaggerated claims of global need in autism have been reduced to a subgroup, sometimes a pretty small group of individuals, where extraordinary benefit has been validated with scrutiny and rigor. Please realize that if we could prevent or cure autism with a vitamin or with all the vitamins used together, then autism would be a trivial problem. It's certainly not.

Is there a vitamin that your autistic child or family member could benefit from? With very strong odds, I can say yes. According to the ARI Parent Responses Tally (ARI Publication 34, 2009), we have the following data –

Vitamin	# of Reports	% Better Behavior	% No Effect	% Worse Behavior
Subcutaneous B_{12}*	899	72	22	6
Oral B_{12}**	98	61	32	7
Cod liver oil, Vitamins A and D	2250	55	41	4
B_6 with magnesium	7556	49	46	4
P5P	920	48	40	11
Vitamin C	3077	46	52	2
Folic Acid	2565	45	50	5
Vitamin A	1535	44	54	3

* From ARI Publ 34 of Feb 2008; oral B_{12} responses are not compiled after that date. Of course, injected B_{12} in any form is not a nutritional supplement; it's a medical intervention with a doctor-prescribed form of B_{12} (injectable methylcobalamin).
** These responses are anecdotal; they are not controlled studies; there is no assurance of a medical diagnosis of autism or ASD for the person taking the vitamin.

Any behavior that seems improved to the parents qualifies the vitamin for a score of "better behavior". But from our perspective, that can be a big plus! There is the aspect that parents are more sensitive and precise umpires of improvement than are the metric tests.

Vitamins and Individuality

We don't have to rack our brains on this. There are lots of predisposing genetic imperfections and varying gene expressions in the ASD population. The nutritional status varies from individual to individual, and the provoking insults may be toxicants, infections, or iatrogenic in nature. And, by iatrogenic, I don't necessarily mean vaccinations at the wrong time. I'd be just as concerned about excessive use of antibiotic medications and pathogenic gut conditions where bad, obstinate microflora take over.

In summary, there are many autisms in the spectrum of autistic disorder. The nutritional regimen that helped Jimmy down the street may not work at all for your family member. That means, you're going to have to do trials of different vitamins and blends of vitamins to find out what works best in your case. My experience tells me that use of a complete blend of vitamins ("multivitamins") usually gives the best results. For some, there can be enhanced benefit with extra amounts of one or two particular vitamins. Some brands already come formulated that way – with increased B_6 and added P5P, for example. That makes life simpler if it works.

Vitamin Tests (Optional Reading)

One strategy that addresses individuality and that may reduce the try-and-see aspect of what vitamin(s) are especially needed is vitamin assay – analytical measurement of vitamins in blood, cells, or urine by a clinical laboratory. Generally, this requires a doctor's order, and the results may come with informative commentary. You should discuss the merits of doing such tests with your doctor and/or nutrition counselor ahead of time. Many times in my experience, vitamin supplements have been notably helpful despite "all normal" analytical results on a laboratory report. Vitamin chemistry in the body is complicated and measured levels of just one vitamer form in one tissue/fluid can be as deceptive as judging a book by reading just one page.

Analytical tests (laboratory tests) for vitamins come in two general varieties, quantitative and functional. Neither is foolproof and neither is able to really test nutritional adequacy of any vitamin. The value of either test is that if a subnormal result is measured, then there is analytical justification for supplementing the vitamin that corresponds to that result.

Quantitative Assays

Quantitative vitamin analysis (assay) is measurement of the concentration of a vitamin in a body fluid or tissue, such as blood plasma, cells, or urine. Measurement units like nanograms or picograms per milliliter of fluid are used and compared with a laboratory reference range. Reference ranges, by the way, are supposed to be established and validated by individual laboratories for each analyte they measure and report.

Using vitamin B_{12} as an example, a normal quantitative result might be 700 picograms per ml of blood serum, with a typical reference range of 350 to 1000 picograms/ml. Below 350 would be low; above 1000 would be high. There are at least two shortcomings with this type of test. The first is, what form of vitamin B_{12} was tested? Not methylcobalamin, the coenzyme form in cell cytosol that assists methionine metabolism. Certainly not adenosylcobalamin, the mitochondrial coenzyme form that assists propionate and methylmalonate chemistry. Depending on the specific analysis technique, what's measured are the in-transport cobalamins. That is, nonfunctional vitamin B_{12} bound to several different carrier proteins or "transcobalamins" are what is measured. So there is no measurement of specific functional forms (coenzyme forms) of the vitamin when we do a quantitative vitamin assay. The second drawback is, of course, that we don't have a measurement of how well the vitamin is working. There would have to be special analyses of what the vitamin does as a coenzyme to find out.

This doesn't mean that quantitative vitamin assay tests are no good. On the contrary, they're good for screening for gross deficiencies – the kind that do occur in this age of processed-food and junk-food diets. Also, there's no practical alternative to quantitative assay of some vitamins, particularly the lipid (oil) soluble ones – vitamins A, D and E. Some of the functions of these nutrients are complex, hormone-like and not easy to single out.

Also, vitamin C (water-soluble) can be quantitatively assayed for its active or chemically-reduced form. One way to do this is with urine analysis. There should be some active vitamin C left over from body needs, which means we would find some active vitamin C in the urine. If there's none, then it's very likely that body tissues ran out of it, and only oxidized vitamin C is left. No – or very little – reduced vitamin C in urine is a sign that more dietary/supplemental vitamin C is needed. In that case, it is likely that other antioxidant nutrients are in short supply too.

Functional Assays

This leads us to functional vitamin analysis, which seemed like the gold standard of vitamin testing 20 years ago. My enthusiasm for it has waned with time and experience.

Urine MMA Assay

Let's continue with vitamin B_{12} as our example. One functional test for adequacy of mitochondrial vitamin B_{12} (adenosylcobalamin) is measurement of urine methylmalonic acid, "MMA". This is an excellent test and one of the few that actually assesses a little bit of what's going on inside cell mitochondria. My polling of doctors at DAN! Think Tanks has led to the conclusion that about 25% of their autistic patient populations had urine MMA above the testing laboratory's reference range. This apparently is typical for new, untreated patients presenting with ASD.

In mitochondria, coenzyme B_{12} assists with a metabolite that comes naturally from the body's use of three nutritionally essential amino acids, methionine, valine and isoleucine. That metabolite, methylmalonic acid, abbreviated "MMA", is supposed to be converted to succinate for citric acid cycle use. That's what adenosylcobalamin assists with. The three amino acids undergo different transformation journeys in body tissues, but all three eventually contribute to formation of propionic acid inside cell mitochondria. Some propionic acid is removed by L-carnitine, and the rest becomes MMA. Then adenosylcobalamin is needed to help change that into succinic acid. If mitochondrial B_{12} isn't able to do its job well enough, excess MMA winds up in the urine. Measuring the urine level of MMA tells us whether vitamin B_{12} as coenzyme adenosylcobalamin is doing an adequate job (well, kind of – read on).

There are two confounding factors that I've learned about for the urine MMA-B_{12} adequacy test. The first is that L-carnitine gets first crack at mitochondrial propionic acid before it's changed into MMA.

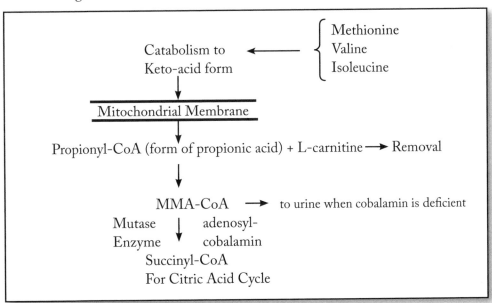

If carnitine is deficient, you might give B_{12} with a wheelbarrow and still have excessive MMA spilling in the urine. The second dilemma is oxidant stress. B_{12} in cells has to be combined with glutathione before it can cross into mitochondria. Once inside, a mitochondrial reductase enzyme has to reduce the oxidation state (valence) of the cobalt in the cobalamin before adenosylcobalamin can be formed. If oxidant stress is really what's preventing B_{12} from doing its mitochondrial job, then antioxidant supplements could be a lot more helpful than more B_{12}.

In general, what else is problematic with functional vitamin assays? It's the limitation that a functional test looks at only one specific function. Luckily, B_{12} has only two important functions in humans. The other one, the cytosolic one, is assisting the recycle of some homocysteine back to methionine – that's what methylcobalamin does. If homocysteine is high in blood or urine, then maybe B_{12} is deficient as methylcobalamin – maybe. Elevated homocysteine can also be due to: vitamin B_6 deficiency or P5P coenzyme dysfunction, folate deficiency or dysfunction (some of which may be genetically based), oxidant stress (which also hinders methylcobalamin's work), or, in rare cases, problems with the next amino acid down the line, cystathionine. The take-home here is that vitamins typically have multiple functions in the body. Testing one function might tell us that something is wrong, or we might miss the real problem and think all is okay when it's really not.

Let me repeat this so there's no misunderstanding. Urine MMA measurement is a good analytical test for an individual with ASD. But an abnormal result is not necessarily going to be remedied by supplementing just vitamin B_{12} (in any form). And a normal result doesn't tell us that the other function of B_{12} is okay.

Urine FIGlu Test

No, this isn't a joke. FIGlu stands for a type of glutamic acid – formiminoglutamic acid. It's glutamic acid with a fancy little carbon and nitrogen piece attached (-CH=NH for you inquisitive chemists). FIGlu comes from histidine, a dietary-source amino acid. Activated (meaning chemically reduced) folic acid, is tetrahydrofolate (THF); that's folate carrying four hydrogen atoms. THF is a receptor for the formimino part of FIGlu; it becomes formimino-THF. That form of folate becomes 5,10-methenyl-THF, which goes through one more transformation before it contributes to assembly of the important nucleosides inosine and adenosine. Sorry about the chemistry, but some of you are bound to ask what FIGlu does. It contributes to adenosine supplies, some of which become ATP, without which we'd be dead – quickly.

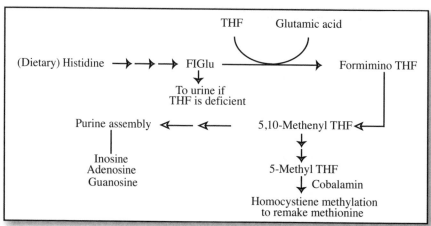

126

Why am I bringing up this perplexing bit of human biochemistry? Because doctors at four DAN! Think Tanks have agreed that between 60% and 80% of their new, untreated ASD patients have mildly elevated urine FIGlu when first tested. These results have come mostly from two clinical laboratories: Genova Diagnostics of Asheville, NC, and MetaMetrix of Norcross, GA. The "highs" are versus laboratory norms, and I believe that both laboratories have independently established pediatric reference ranges for urine FIGlu.

Reference to almost any physiology or laboratory analysis textbook will tell you that high urine FIGlu means inadequate folate activity as THF. Well, not quite. The second edition of Howerde Sauberlich's outstanding text: Laboratory Tests for the Assessment of Nutritional Status, CRC Press (1999) says vitamin B_{12} problems can also cause a high FIGlu result (page 122). Then, there's the fact that the enzyme that transfers the formimino piece from glutamate to THF needs P5P as a coenzyme (P5P, or pyridoxal 5-phosphate, comes from vitamin B_6.) And, the enzyme is part of a microtubular protein structure in cells (in Golgi complexes) which are relatively fragile, possibly damaged by toxicant chemicals. And, per the doctors at the DAN! Think Tanks, folate supplements sometimes do not significantly improve the urine FIGlu excess. Instead, these doctors say that vitamin B_{12} and detoxification therapies often result in normalization of urine FIGlu levels. Occasionally, nothing they've tried helps.

The take-home here is that, while urine FIGlu often is mildly elevated in urine from autistics (mostly children), giving folate is frequently not the answer. Something else is wrong in most cases. Maybe the body doesn't want any more adenosine and there is some feedback regulation of the formiminoTHF precursor assembly line? This is a tough problem, and we don't have it figured out.

Where does that leave us with vitamin testing? We know that if a vitamin assay, quantitative or functional, shows a deficiency, then there's something wrong, but supplementing the vitamin isn't a sure fix. We also know that a "normal" result can be truly meaningless, especially for a quantitative test. Quantitative tests don't show how well or how poorly the vitamin is working. That's why giving complete vitamin blends, balanced or enhanced in certain ways, makes the most sense when intervening nutritionally in ASD. It's also why you're typically going to do try-and-see trials with vitamin blends and perhaps specific vitamins given in addition to the blend or multivitamin supplement.

Vitamin Data

Before launching into descriptions of the vitamins, let's understand some basics about use of nutritional products and product labels.

Using Safe Amounts

Safety is always an issue and there's always such a thing as too much. In college, I joined the chemistry fraternity, Alpha Chi Sigma. The historic mentor of this fraternity is the Swiss physician (and alchemist) Paracelsus who lived 500 years ago. Attributed to him is the concept that "everything is poisonous, it's just a matter of amount."

When we refer to medical or physiology textbooks for overdose levels of vitamins, we find that schedule of use (acute or chronic) is an issue. Scientific papers and toxicology texts tell us that purity and vitamer form also are issues. When we read nutrition texts, we find that some chemicals in the body can protect if they're adequate. Taurine, for example, helps to dispose of used, excess vitamin A. In other words, individuality contributes to the safety issue.

As a general rule for use of vitamins and for all nutritional supplements, start at low amounts and work upward while watching for effects, good and bad. Supplement products, by law, have a daily serving amount on the label. Confer with your doctor or nutrition counselor before exceeding that amount, or don't exceed it.

Product Labels, Amounts and Percentages

There's a mystery out there, one with a title that keeps changing – "Recommended Dietary Allowance" (RDA), "Recommended Daily Intake" (RDI), "Dietary Reference Intake" (DRI), "Daily Value", "% of Daily Value", etc. What's going on here? Historically, the Food and Nutrition Board of the US National Research Council established (or postulated) that certain amounts of vitamins in the diet are necessary to prevent disease in a healthy human population. Those postulated amounts are a function of age and sex. A thorough description of this effort is published: National Research Council, *Recommended Dietary Allowances*, 10th Edition, National Academy Press (1989). More recently, responsibility for recommendations on nutritional intake rests with a committee of the Food and Nutrition Board of the Institute of Medicine (IOM).

Such amounts of essential nutrients by any name do not guarantee nutritional adequacy for any individual – nor would amounts ten times higher. RDAs and similar compilations of RDIs and DRIs apply to a healthy population and not to individuals with particular problems in metabolism. Those with metabolic problems, inherited or acquired, might benefit from considerably more of a certain nutrient.

We run into a special version of these recommended amounts whenever we purchase a container of supplements that includes some of the codified nutrients – vitamins, essential minerals (elements), perhaps protein, etc. This special version of the amounts is set by the Food and Drug Administration (FDA). The FDA amounts are legal reference levels and are not a function of age or sex. They are codified in FDA regulations (21 CFR Chapter1). They rarely, if ever, change. The FDA reference levels are typical of adult RDA/RDI/DRI amounts; they are not children's amounts, even if the supplement product is intended for children. For example, the National Research Council set these RDAs for vitamin B_6 in milligrams/day: children 1-3 yrs, 0.5; children 4-8 yrs, 0.6; males 14-18 yrs, 1.3; females 14-18 yrs 1.2; males 51-70 yrs 1.7, pregnant women 10-30 yrs, 1.9 during lactation 2.0; women 51-70 yrs 1.5. The FDA reference level ("Daily Value") is simply 2.0 mg/day. Tabulated below are some FDA reference levels (formerly, "US RDAs", currently "Daily Values").

FDA Reference Levels for Essential Nutrients

Vitamin A	5000 IU
Vitamin C	60 mg
Vitamin D	400 IU
Vitamin E	30 IU
Thiamine (B$_1$)	1.5 mg
Riboflavin (B$_2$)	1.7 mg
Niacin (B$_3$)	20 mg
Pyridoxine (B$_6$)	2.0 mg
Vitamin B$_{12)}$	6 micrograms
Pantothenic acid	10 mg
Folic acid	0.4 mg (400 micrograms)
Calcium	1.0 gram (1000 mg)
Magnesium	400 mg
Iodine	150 micrograms
Iron	18 mg
Zinc	15 mg

I'm often asked, "How long does a vitamin last in the body?" That's also an individual issue as is "How much is appropriate?" The Vitamin Data Table that follows compiles some of that information.

VITAMIN DATA TABLE, 2011

Vitamin	Half-Life In humans	Units and conversions	Supplement Range (oral)	Chronic use overdose levels oral
Vitamin A, Retinol	3-6 weeks	Biopotency: 3.33×10^3 IU/mg 1.0 USP unit = 0.30µg of retinol = 0.344µg of vitamin A acetate	1000-10,000 IU/d	> 50,000 IU/d >15 to 20 mg/d depends on taurine status, biliary fctn.
Beta-carotene	controlled conversion to retinol	1 IU = 0.6 µg B-carotene	2000-20,000 IU/D	Carotenemia at > 50,000 IU/d; does NOT cause hypervitaminosis A
B_1, thiamin	~ 1 day	1 USP unit = 3µg Of thiamin•HCl	10-100 mg/d	< 125 mg/kg body weight
B_2, riboflavin	4-5 days	1000 µg = 1 mg	5-50 mg/d	unknown in humans
B_3, niacin	1-2 days	1000 µg = 1 mg	niacin, 20-100 mg/d niacinamide, 50-1000 mg/d	>100 mg causes skin flushing; no flushing with nicotinamide (niacinamide)
Pantothenate	~2 days	1000 µg = 1 mg	10-100 mg/d	unknown in humans
B_6, pyridoxine	~ 1 day	1000 µg = 1 mg	B_6, 10-100 mg/d P5P, 5-50 mg/d	B_6 > 500 mg/day may induce (reversible) peripheral neuropathy
B_{12}, cobalamin	350-400 days	1000 µg = 1 mg 1 USP unit = 1 µg (cyanocobalamin)	50-5000 µg/d	unknown in humans, cobalt not toxic as cobalamin
Folic acid	~ 1 day	1000 µg = 1 mg	200-1000 µg/d	unknown in humans
Biotin	2-6 weeks	1000 µg = 1 mg	100-1000 µg/d	unknown in humans
Vitamin C Ascorbic acid	16 days	1000 mg + 1 g	50-200 mg/d	urinary mineral loss w/ ascorbic acid > 4000 mg/d
Vitamin D	1-3 weeks	1 µg D_2 = 40 USP units 0.025 µg D_3 = 1 USP unit 1 USP unit = 1 IU	200-1200 IU/d	form and calcium status dependent, > 2000 IU/d D_3
Vitamin E	12-15 days	1 mg d-α-E = 1.49 IU 1 mg d,l-α-E = 1.0 IU	30-400 IU/d	anticoagulant potential if E > 1000 IU/d

Explanatory Notes to Vitamin Data Table

Half-Life: the biologic half-life or the time period during which one half of the vitamin is "used up", or excreted; at that point one half still remains in body tissues. Of course, this assumes that there is no additional input of the vitamin during the half-life period. These half-lives do not necessarily apply to megadosing. With megadosing, the first one or two half-lives may be considerably different, usually shorter. Further, the half-lives are averages or calculated averages for normal, healthy individuals. Biochemical and metabolic individuality, stress and disease would be expected to alter these half-lives for a specific individual.

Megadosing: is supplementation at a level considerably above the US government-established levels that are deemed necessary to prevent disease in a healthy human population. Megadosing may be appropriate to address a disease condition for which elevated levels of the vitamin or its cofactor metabolite are considered beneficial.

Units and Conversions: mg = milligram, one-thousandth of a gram; ug, μg or mcg = microgram, one-millionth of a gram.

Supplement Range: the daily oral amount that is found in various vitamin supplements that I believe to be appropriate for many with ASD. The supplement amounts range to levels above the "Daily Value" in order to –

        a) Potentiate an enzyme or enzymes that are dysfunctional or weak and depend upon the coenzyme form of the vitamin for their biochemical activity.

        b) Overcome renal loss in a renal wasting condition,

        c) Overcome poor uptake due to an intestinal malabsorption condition,

        d) Combat infections,

        e) Combat chemical toxicity, enhance enzymatic detoxication processes, or provide enhanced antioxidant capability.

The lower levels should be used for children. Megadose levels (amounts above the supplement range) should be under a doctor's supervision. If the supplement range exceeds the label-posted daily serving amounts, I recommend conferring with your doctor or nutrition counselor before using such amounts.

Overdose Levels: amounts at or above these levels could provoke symptoms or side effects depending on biochemical individuality. In most cases, the symptoms are reversible by lowering or discontinuing the vitamin intake. More information on overdose levels can be found in *Drug Facts and Comparisons*, Wolter Kluwer Health, St. Louis, MO.

While niacinamide (and inositol hexanicotinate) may be used in megadose quantities (1000 mg and above), this is NOT suggested for ASD. Megadose B_3 in any form causes loss of methylation capacity via urinary loss of methylnicotinamide.

Oral Use of the B-Vitamins and Folate for ASD

These vitamins are –

B_1, thiamine (or thiamin)

B_2, riboflavin

B_3, niacin

B_6, pyridoxine

B_{12}, cobalamin

Pantothenate (no, it's not "B_5")

Folic acid

All of these vitamins dissolve somewhat readily in water, making them quite bioavailable but also subject to short residence times in our bodies. An exception is B_{12}, which has a rather complicated uptake mechanism and very long residence time.

B_1 is often stabilized as the mononitrate or hydrochloride; either is fine at supplemental levels.

B_3 often is provided in the nonflushing (skin) form, niacinamide, or even better, inositol hexanicotinate, which also provides a near-vitamin nutrient and growth factor, inositol.

B_6 is typically sold in the stabilized form pyridoxine·HCl (hydrochloride), also safe at supplemental levels although acidic. Providing some B_6 in the actual coenzyme form, pyridoxal 5-phosphate, gets past the pyridoxine $\rightarrow$ pyridoxal hurdle of coenzyme formation even though the phosphate part is lost during uptake from the intestinal tract (it's replaced inside cells). Providing B_6 as 80-90% pyridoxine and 10-20% pyridoxal phosphate especially benefits a subset of ASD individuals.

Pantothenic acid is usually provided as calcium pantothenate, a stabilized form of that vitamin.

B_{12} generally is sold in the stabilized forms – cyanocobalamin. This is a microgram-quantity nutrient, and the cyano part (cyanide-related) is easily handled by either the body's enzymatic detoxication capability (rhodanase, which makes thiocyanate) or by alpha-ketoglutaric acid, the tissue levels of which can combine with and eliminate trace cyanide with negligible depletion. Also, it is a good idea to provide some vitamin B_{12} as methylcobalamin, especially when methylation chemistry might be inhibited, as clinical research indicates is the case for many with ASD. Its stability is markedly less than that of cyanocobalamin, so when you use this form, keep the container dark, cool, and tightly closed.

Use of coenzyme forms of vitamins B_1 or B_2 is problematic with conflicting reports on benefit. These forms are thiamine diphosphate, riboflavin monophosphate or mononucleotide (FMN), or flavin adenine dinucleotide (FAD). They are not well assimilated into blood from the gastrointestinal tract; to be absorbed they have to be dephosphorylated (disassembled). Unlike B_6, nothing is gained from oral use of coenzyme forms of B_1 or B_2, and it's likely that these forms make the body's nutritional uptake job harder.

Generally, we don't use these vitamins separately because they work much better when there is a cooperative effort. It's true that nutritional therapy for autism began with use of vitamin B_6, and there are 22 published articles attesting to that. Twenty-one of the 22 reported beneficial results. Purists, however, find fault with just about all of these studies due to lack of proper controls, lack of rigorous measurement metrics for judging improvement, small sample size (not enough subjects), other interfering goings-on, etc.

On grounds of biochemistry, I don't like giving just vitamin B_6, or any single vitamin. Here's why, using B_6 as the example. First, B_6 as pyridoxine has to be oxidized to pyridoxal, an enzymatic step enhanced by a coenzyme form of riboflavin, flavin mononucleotide (FMN). To make FMN from riboflavin, magnesium is required as an enzyme activator, as is phosphate from ATP. Next, the pyridoxal needs phosphate, also from ATP. A zinc-promoted enzyme (pyridoxal kinase) handles that. Inside cells when more pyridoxal phosphate is needed, what gives the signals? Melatonin does. After all this happens, P5P is ready to work. But you know what? A plentiful amount of P5P can interfere with a detoxication process called sulfation. This was studied and reported on to ARI by Dr. Rosemary Waring, Birmingham University, UK. However, magnesium supplements accelerate the sulfation step with which pyridoxal competes. Magnesium is a balancing, synergistic nutrient that has to be used along with vitamin B_6 for many individuals with ASD.

Now, how far are we going to get if we supplement only pyridoxine and not riboflavin, magnesium, zinc, melatonin, etc? To find that out, we have to look at older editions of ARI Publication 34, one published prior to 1995, because ARI stopped correlating single B_6 results when parents stopped using it singly. Fewer than 30% were helped, with about 10% having worse behavior (n~600).

What have parents reported about using B_6 plus magnesium? 49% better and only 4% worse. And melatonin gets 66% improved. The take-home here is that we're going to use groups of supplements at various stages of intervention, and it's best to use multivitamin blends that contain assisting and synergistic nutrients. And when certain assisting nutrients are not included in the blends (such as melatonin or taurine, not usually included in multivitamins), it makes sense to add those to the regimen. See Supplement Intervention Schedule.

B-Vitamin Benefits for ASD (Optional Reading)

If you're interested in learning all about what vitamins do, this isn't the place. Please refer to the publications listed in Literature-Vitamins at the end of this section. There are quite a few books that provide lay information about vitamins and other nutrients; also listed there are physiology and biochemistry books for more advanced interests. **Here, I'm confining the text to why I think these vitamins can be beneficial to individuals with ASD. Occasionally this gets technical, and you don't need to know all of this to do nutritional intervention. I've provided this information because experience has taught me that some of you do want it.**

About Thiamine (Optional Reading)

There are two parts of physiology that clinicians and biochemistry researchers believe to be in trouble for some with ASD and that are thiamine-related:

1. Making enough of the very important antioxidant cofactor, NADPH, a coenzyme form of niacin (B_3),
2. Getting enough energy (as ATP) from mitochondrial processes.

(1) In our tissues, much of the chemistry that balances the oxidation-reduction that's always occurring comes from glucose which originates from dietary carbohydrates. From research I did thirty years ago, through to the work of many others today, oxidant stress has

been identified as a physiologic problem in many with ASD. Oxidant stress is an excess of reactive chemicals in cells and tissues. Oxidant damage and inflammation occur when these chemicals react with cell membranes, proteins, or with other normal metabolites, and oxidize them.

One thing that sugar (as glucose 6-phosphate) is supposed to do is allow hydrogen to be added to the phosphorylated, coenzyme form of vitamin B_3, nicotinamide adenine dinucleotide; it's denoted "NADP".

$$NADP + H \rightarrow NADPH.$$

This loading of hydrogen onto coenzyme B_3 costs energy, releases CO_2, and changes the chemical form of the sugar molecule. Central to this process is the vitamin B_1 as coenzyme thiamine diphosphate. Without thiamine diphosphate it isn't possible to use sugar to make NADPH. The sugar becomes ribose, and that's used to make nucleic acid and nucleotides. If you wish to learn more about this process, look up the "hexose monophosphate shunt" in a physiology or biochemistry book.

NADPH is the top-grade carrier of antioxidant hydrogen which it can give away to regenerate the other antioxidant workers in our tissues. For example, NADPH feeds hydrogen to glutathione reductase for enzymatic regeneration of glutathione (GSH).

$$GSSG \text{ (oxidized)} + 2 \text{ NADPH} \rightarrow 2 \text{ GSH (reduced, active)} + 2 \text{ NADP}$$

Subnormal NADPH in some with autism is a research finding by Tapan Audhya, Ph.D., presented at DAN! Think Tanks by associated researcher, James Adams, Ph.D. (Arizona State U). This finding was also presented at the Annual Autism/Asperger's Conference, Phoenix, 2008, by Dr. Audhya. As of that date, there were 52 control children and 127 tested autistics in the study. Control erythrocyte NADPH ranged from 24.5 to 49.6 nanomoles/ml (37.8 mean), and 78 of the autistics had significantly lowered NADPH levels, 8.3 to 20.4 (11.7 mean). A distinct group of forty nine autistic study subjects had essentially normal NADPH levels.

(2) Are you ready for the second ASD-benefit from thiamine? That benefit is getting more ATP made by getting more energy conversions working in cell mitochondria. For those with interest and experience in biochemistry, the areas of concern are the pyruvate dehydrogenase complex, the citric acid cycle, and phosphorylation in the mitochondrial respiratory chain.

For the rest of us, here's what is going on. Carbohydrates and some amino acids are processed into pyruvate, a simple carbohydrate. With amino acids, this requires nitrogen (amino group) removal – that's mostly done by vitamin B_6 as P5P assisting a family of enzymes called transaminases. (There will be more about that in the pyridoxine section.) Pyruvate is allowed passage through the mitochondrial membranes; its precursors, stuff like fructose, glucose, and glycerate, can't get in. Once inside, most of the pyruvate is changed into chemical fuel for energy transfer chemistry (called the "citric acid cycle"). The enzyme system that changes pyruvate to fuel is called the "pyruvate dehydrogenase complex", PDH.

PDH uses thiamine diphosphate as well as a riboflavin coenzyme, FAD, and lipoate (lipoic acid). The workings of PDH are shut down by mercury, arsenic, and possibly by other toxicants. When PDH inhibition occurs, as you'd expect, pyruvate accumulates and blood/urine levels go up. This is seen in some with ASD. Elevations of pyruvate, alanine (formed from pyruvate), lactate, and perhaps the branched-chain amino acids (valine, leucine, isoleucine) can be markers for inhibited PDH, and supplemental thiamine is one possible remedy (Harper's Review of Biochemistry, 20th Ed).

The take home: thiamine is necessary as part of the vitamin team for ASD. Daily amounts of 5 to 100 mg often are offered in different supplement products. My experience is that 10 to 25 mg/day is plenty when the rest of the vitamin team is present. More can be beneficial in special cases, when your doctor so directs.

About Riboflavin (Optional Reading)

We met one of riboflavin's coenzyme activities earlier in the vitamin teamwork discussion. It accelerates the formation of P5P from pyridoxine. It is true that P5P can be formed in our cells without riboflavin's help as FMN, flavin mononucleotide, but the rate of formation then is slow. What else is riboflavin needed for?

In mitochondria, the citric acid cycle and subsequent energy transfer processes need FAD to make ADP (which becomes ATP). FAD is the other cofactor/coenzyme that riboflavin makes – flavin adenine dinucleotide (made of riboflavin, two phosphates, ribose sugar and adenine). While we're on energy supply, there's another important mitochondrial role for riboflavin as FAD. This is the enzyme that promotes the first step of fatty acid oxidation – a major energy-supply process that enables mitochondrial function.

Riboflavin also helps us detoxify. Aldehydes are chemicals similar to organic acids; they're made naturally in cells but can also result from contaminations in our environment. Yeast overgrowth in the gut can result in uptake of acetaldehyde, which can have toxic consequences. There's a detoxifying enzyme for aldehydes that's mostly active in liver tissue – aldehyde dehydrogenase. It's FAD-dependent.

Obviously, riboflavin is a very necessary part of the vitamin team, and amounts of 5 to 50 mg/d are appropriate. Children usually don't need more than 10 to 20 mg/d.. It has a yellow pigment property, and yellow-colored urine means it was absorbed and there's some left. That's fine. Medical and biochemistry reference books say that toxic levels of riboflavin are unknown in humans (provided that kidney function is normal). The body excretes what isn't needed.

About Niacin, Inositol and Choline (Optional Reading)

Chemists call niacin, nicotinic acid. If diets are supplemented with more than 25-50 mg (children), or 50-100 mg (adults), the skin "flushes", a reddish hue with a warm sensation. If the amide form is used (an amide is nitrogen plus hydrogen), where the amide substitutes for the acid part of the vitamin molecule, we have nicotinamide, and skin flushing does not occur.

There is another non-flushing form, too, inositol hexanicotinate. That molecule is six niacins attached to one inositol, and the special perk is inclusion of cell growth-factor inositol - not strictly a vitamin for humans, but almost! Inositol is a natural food substance that facilitates cell growth. Under normal circumstances, it is also made in our bodies and, as far as I know, is present in every healthy cell. Some animals need it, and for them, it's a vitamin. In mice, for example, absolute dietary deprivation of inositol results in loss of hair, ocular disorders, poor growth and failure to lactate.

Like choline, inositol beneficially influences fatty acid metabolism. Like choline, we make it and also get some from the diet. Like choline, it has always been "conditionally essential" and not-quite-qualified to be a vitamin. But guess what – after decades of being a second-class nutrient, choline was formally promoted to essential status in April of 1998. That hasn't happened yet for inositol.

Niacin forms two absolutely necessary cofactor/coenzyme forms which include adenine, NADH (H, hydrogen, makes it the active, reduced form) and NADPH (contains phosphate as well). NADPH was discussed earlier – it uses energy from sugar to get its hydrogen and then it donates that hydrogen to keep some important antioxidant, anti-inflammatory chemistry working – notably that of glutathione.

What does NADH do? Pretty much the same thing, except it's used where the special phosphate version isn't needed. That doesn't mean it's less important. Mitochondria in cells would burn themselves up without NADH. But neither NADH nor NADPH can cross the double membrane barrier that protects mitochondrial processes. Energy dynamics that occur inside need more hydrogen quench than is internally available, and our cells have evolved with an external supply of antioxidant hydrogen from NADH without letting NADH itself enter.

What happens is that cytosolic NADH gives its H to oxaloacetic acid which is made in the cytosol. Oxaloacetic acid + hydrogen makes malic acid, and malate is allowed into mitochondria. Once inside, it finds NAD in need of hydrogen and it reverses the outside process. Malate becomes oxaloacetic acid and NAD gets its hydrogen, making NADH. Oxaloacetate finds glutamate, makes alpha-ketoglutarate, which has a universal passport and goes out to the cytosol. There it is transformed back to oxaloacetate. This whole transport process, getting hydrogen from NADH into a mitochondrion, is called "the malate shuttle".

My experience is that ASD children do best when little or no nicotinic acid is supplemented, but do quite well with modest amounts of nicotinamide and inositol nicotinate. Total supplemental amounts of either or both of 20 to 100 (max) mg/d can be appropriate, but not more. NADH has also become available as a supplement. I've heard some good reports about it – so far, all anecdotal, but promising.

Larger amounts of vitamin B_3 have been taken under medical supervision for conditions other than ASD. Megadose quantities (1000 to 5000 mg/d) have been successfully used to alleviate some types of schizophrenia. Here, the physiologic objective is to reduce methyl groups. This is opposite to that of ASD therapy, which seeks to increase methylation of homocysteine and increase quantities of substances made by methylation: carnitine, creatine and melatonin. With some types of schizophrenia, removal of methyls leads to improvement. Vitamin B_3 works toward this end by forming its waste metabolite N-methylnicotinamide, which is excreted in the urine. In other words, each molecule of vitamin B_3, when we're done with it, leaves the body with one methyl attached. Vitamin B_3 is needed on the supplement team, but in relatively small amounts. Supplements exceeding a few hundred milligrams of B_3/day can be detrimental if they deplete the methyl supply.

About Pyridoxine, P5P and Magnesium

Pyridoxine is vitamin B_6 and pyridoxal 5-phosphate (P5P) is the active coenzyme form. Vitamin B_6 is the grandfather of nutritional supplements reported by parents and many clinicians to improve autistic traits and behaviors. The first clinical study on pyridoxine use occurred in 1965 (Drs. Heeley and Roberts, *Dev Med Child Neurol* 3:1966, 708-18). They gave one-time doses of 30 mg pyridoxine to 16 autistic children. There was no control group, and the biochemical effect was measured by also giving an oral challenge of the essential amino acid tryptophan, whose metabolism is B_6-dependent. When vitamin B_6 is insufficient, tryptophan metabolism slows down and urine excretion of several telltale metabolites increases. These telltale markers can be measured by laboratory analysis. An oral load of tryptophan accentuates these telltale signs of B_6 insufficiency. Then, giving some amount of B_6 shows whether or not it is beneficial for tryptophan metabolism. Eleven of the 16 children showed normalization of tryptophan metabolism after the pyridoxine dose, five did not. One child was continued on daily B_6 supplements and was reported to have made "remarkable" behavioral progress.

Through the years, many more tests of vitamin B_6 supplements for autism and ASD were performed. You can obtain a summary from ARI of the 22 vitamin B_6 trials that were done by various investigators from 1965 to 2003. The title of the ARI summary is "Studies of High Dosage Vitamin B_6 (and Often with Magnesium) In Autistic Children and Adults". It is five pages by hard copy; available on the website www.autism.com. Twenty-one of these tests reflect beneficial outcomes. Recently, several more vitamin B_6 studies have been published by Professor James Adams, R. Tapan Audhya, and others. These are also available at that website. The new studies show the complexity of trying to assess what's going on with pyridoxine, pyridoxal, phosphorylation and P5P levels in blood versus levels in cells.

During the last 45 years, some of the trials involved increasing doses of pyridoxine – all the way up to the range of 500 to 1125 mg/day (Lelord, 1981). In the early 1980s, Chris and I were directed to use 500 mg/d pyridoxine with our son. The outcome was not good. After a week he showed nervousness and increased agitation, and we chose to discontinue that amount. We went back to 50 mg (along with other B-vitamins at moderate supplemental levels) and he stayed there with good results.

As with any supplemental nutrient, there's a quantity issue due to trace impurities. In 1987, a highly publicized clinical study documented sensory neuropathy with continued oral use of megadose pyridoxine ([Dalton and Dalton] *Acto Neurol Scand* 76 (1987) 8-11). The Dalton's study included about 170 women and the associated daily supplemented pyridoxine intakes varied from below 50 mg up to 500. The syndrome reported by the Daltons included numbness in arms and legs, bone pain, muscle weakness and paresthesias (sensations of tingling, prickling or burning). Pyridoxine got 100% of the blame.

In subsequent studies (with no fanfare or publicity), interfering vitamers were identified as contaminants that may or may not be present in batches of manufactured pyridoxine. To a great extent, vitamin manufacturers cleaned up their acts between 1990 and 2000. Now, however, with all of the foreign-sourced ingredients, I'm again concerned, and I fully support a policy of having detailed analyses for purity provided by the manufacturer.

During much the same period of time, clinicians learned that magnesium needs to be taken along with pyridoxine or pyridoxal phosphate (which is absorbed into the

blood as pyridoxal with phosphate being replaced later inside cells). **If magnesium isn't taken at the same time, extra pyridoxal can interfere with enzyme activity that promotes sulfation. Sulfation is the addition of sulfate to molecules to change their function or to make them water soluble for detoxication and excretion. This has been studied and documented by Dr. Rosemary Waring, and a report is available from ARI.**

Once again, it's the tally of results that matters most. Per ARI Pub 34 (2009), 49% get better with B_6 + magnesium; only 4% get worse, n=7256.

Because P5P has so many coenzyme roles in human cells and tissue, exactly where it's helping half of the ASD population is conjecture. Probably there's a big variance due to individuality and to the precise biochemical need. Here are some candidate areas in biochemistry where P5P helps out.

1. That malate shuttle I told you about earlier (getting hydrogen for antioxidant uses into mitochondria) – well, it doesn't work without P5P. That's because the shuttle depends upon alpha-ketoglutarate grabbing an amino part from aspartate to become glutamate, etc. Amino transfers use a 'transaminase" enzyme, and transaminases require P5P. So, without P5P, our mitochondria are toast.

2. Transaminase enzymes (lots of different ones) contain the amino acid lysine, and lysine is where the P5P gets attached. But lysine on proteins is where homocysteine thiolactone attaches – the kind of dead-end homocysteine that happens when organophosphates use (and maybe wreck) the homocysteine-rescue enzyme, "paraoxonase". And it's been recently discovered that paraoxonase has great variability in children – so it may or may not be adequate to begin with. For these people, organophosphate contamination could be enough to push a physiologic weakness into a pathologic disaster. Supplemental pyridoxine competes for the lysine attachment site and bolsters transaminase activity.

3. In the metabolic journey that methionine takes to form cysteine and taurine, P5P is required multiple times. Detoxication, antioxidant and anti-inflammatory function, immune response, biliary excretion of wastes and biliary uptake of essential lipids all have some dependence on this metabolic path.

4. Some seizure cases feature an excess of CNS glutamate and a deficiency of gamma-aminobutyric acid (GABA). Glutamate is an excitatory neurotransmitter; GABA is inhibitory. The enzyme that promotes the transformation of glutamate into GABA requires P5P.

5. Tryptophan metabolism is very P5P dependent, including the route to serotonin. Serotonin precedes melatonin, which, when supplemented, helps over 60% with ASD.

Using Vitamin B$_6$ in ASD

During the last decade, many supplement manufacturers reduced the level of vitamin B$_6$ in multivitamins to accommodate the concerns that I mentioned. No longer is 500 mg considered a good idea unless it's under a doctor's direction. Also, with all of the other nutritional team members on board, pyridoxine isn't being asked to do its work alone.

Is magnesium adequate? Here's a table of B$_6$ and magnesium (Mg) requirement and suggested supplement levels as a function of child weight.

Body wt, kilograms	NAS/IOM daily recommended mg,	B$_6$ + P5P max suggested Mg	Additional Mg, mg (at least)
10	80	25	15
20	130	50	30
30	190	50	30
40 and above	260	100	60

Pyridoxine plus P5P in amounts that total over 100 mg should be used under a doctor's direction. This is a cautionary change from what I and others, including the late Dr. Bernard Rimland, said some years ago. There are metabolic disorders for which benefit is derived from pyridoxine supplementation at levels above 100 mg/d, but these are uncommon disorders.

About Pantothenic Acid (Optional Reading)

First of all, let's understand that there's a name problem. Not because it makes a big difference to us, but because a nutritional biochemist or a graduate in nutritional science will think we're uninformed if we call this stuff "vitamin B$_5$". It's really not, though it's sometimes called that, even in some books.

In the 1920s-30s, food science researchers did extensive work to identify the trace ingredients in food that humans can't live without. Vitamin A was identified in 1913 and the next job was to characterize vitamin B. Vitamin B actually was identified in 1910 in Japan by Dr. Suzuki, but we weren't communicating well back then. British chemist Casimir Funk isolated an anti-beriberi factor in 1911 and named it 'vitamine". However, the chemical structure eluded scientists until 1934. By then, they knew that there wasn't just one vitamin B. The Suzuki-Funk factor was first in line, and it got to be Vitamin B$_1$, thiamine.

There were more than a dozen other B-vitamin candidates put forth by various teams of investigators. You know B$_2$ and B$_3$ as riboflavin and niacin. What was B$_4$? It was adenine, which becomes adenosine when ribose sugar is added, and then becomes AMP, ADP, and ATP when phosphates are added to that. Adenine was demoted from vitamin candidate status when we discovered that it is made adequately in cells via "purine" metabolism. What was proposed as B$_5$? It was a growth factor for pigeons, described in a 1930 issue of The Journal of Biochemistry. It didn't make the grade either.

Pantothenate often is called "vitamin B$_5$", and nutritionists will know what you mean when you use the term – but I think you should at least be aware of the facts. Pantothenate was described by Williams et al. in a 1938 issue of the Journal of the American Chemical Society. It gets its name from pantoic acid, which is part of the vitamin structure; the amino acid beta-alanine is the other part. Some gut bacteria can put pantoic acid and beta-alanine together and make the vitamin; humans can't. The problem is, our gut bacteria don't make enough, so some is needed in our food or in supplements. This vitamin is almost always stabilized and provided as calcium D-pantothenate. Pure pantothenate is a viscous, oily substance that is miscible with water and that oxidizes in air at room temperature. The calcium form is solid, can be loaded into capsules as a fine powder, and is water-soluble.

The active form of pantothenate is coenzyme A, "CoA", and making it in the body is very energy intensive – requires four ATPs or three ATPs and one CTP. Synthesis of CoA also requires cysteine, and one of the ATPs has to dump all its phosphates to add its adenosine on. That means we have to make a new adenosine for each CoA that is formed. Precious is the word you should associate with CoA. In some books, it's denoted CoASH where the –SH recognizes the sulfur-hydrogen piece of the cysteine part (analogous to GSH for glutathione). This –SH part is where much of CoA's chemical activity occurs.

CoA is a powerhouse coenzyme. In mitochondria, it is required by the chemistry that makes cellular energy from fats and carbohydrates. Mitochondrial energy conversion processes are dead without it. Making bigger fatty acids from smaller ones requires CoA as well (a cytosolic process). Some of the body's major detoxication processes depend upon CoA, too – acetylation (sulfonamides and sulfa drugs, PABA, benzidine, amines, anilines, aminophenols, unneeded serotonin), bile formation (excretion pathway for all kinds of unwanted stuff), and peptide conjugation of CoA-activated junk (benzoate, phenylacetate).

There's a natural source that's very rich in pantothenate, but you have to go into a beehive to get it. It's the special honey that the queen bee makes, "royal jelly". You might get the regular honey out, but they'll fight you for this stuff. Multivitamin supplements usually include 10 to 50 mg per daily amount or per serving, and amounts of 100 to 200 mg/d can be beneficial for some. Toxicity or overdose does not seem to be an issue for pantothenate.

About Cobalamin (Optional Reading)

Like proposed vitamin B_4 and the original B_5, the trace ingredients in food that were proposed as vitamins B_7-B_{11} didn't make the grade either. The next one in the B sequence to do so was B_{12}, and it's named cobalamin because it contains the metal element cobalt as an activator. Cobalamin (Cbl) achieved vitamin status because it can't be synthesized it in the body, and because researchers found that without it, humans develop anemia and neurological impairments. Isolation of the red-colored crystalline form of B_{12} and declaration of vitamin status occurred in 1944 – Rickes, et al, *Science* 107 (1944) 296. We now add glossitis, fatigue or generalized weakness, mental depression, dementia, and immune deficiency (suppressed natural killer cell activity) to the list of maladies associated with B_{12} deficiency.

In the body, Cbl exists in several chemical forms, but only two coenzyme actions are known –

1) Remethylation of some homocysteine in the cytosol part of cells to remake methionine, which adds to the methionine that's obtained from digestion of dietary protein, and

2) Converting methylmalonic acid, MMA, to succinic acid, which occurs inside cell mitochondria. Actually, MMA has to be attached to coenzyme A for this conversion to occur, so add this to the list of what CoA (from pantothenate) is required for.

Dietary uptake of vitamin B_{12} is a bit complicated, but worth learning about. It starts with the stomach secreting "intrinsic factor", a constituent of gastric juice. B_{12} gets attached to intrinsic factor and carried to the ileum part of the small intestine. One of intrinsic factor's jobs is to protect the B_{12} from digestion, and another is to locate the special microvillae sites on the mucosa of the ileum where B_{12} absorption will take place. Once absorbed, the B_{12} meets its next escort, one of two proteins – "transcobalamin I" or "transcobalamin II", to which most blood plasma Cbl is attached. By now you're probably getting the idea that Cbl is a fragile nutrient that always requires a chaperone. You're right, it does.

If Cbl goes to the liver, the chaperone that holds onto it is transcobalmin I. Other destinations involve transcobalamin II. Once cobalamin reaches a cell where it is eventually to be used, it gets stashed as hydroxocobalamin in the cell's lysosomes. Hydroxocobalamin is a storage form, and the cobalt state is +3 (oxidized, and therefore stable). Lysosomes are tiny compartments in the cytosol region of cells where water-soluble material is kept and processed.

When Cbl is needed for either of its two coenzyme functions, it has to join up with another protective escort, one that we're all familiar with – glutathione (GSH). Together, they become glutathionyl cobalamin, GSCbl. Then a decision has to be made. Is the Cbl going to assist remethylation of homocysteine to form methionine (cytosolic), or is it needed in mitochondria to process MMA?

Most methylation reactions in the body require S-adenosylmethionine, SAM, as the methyl donor. Some important products of SAM methylation are melatonin, creatine, carnitine, methylated phospholipids in neurons adjacent to message receptors, and internally-made choline, which becomes TMG and DMG. SAM is made from methionine and ATP, and the methionine all originates from dietry protein – except that there's an important recycle supply of methionine. After SAM gives away its methyl part, what's left is homocysteine joined to adenosine. After adenosine departs (which can be a big problem for some with autism), we're left with homocysteine. Now, metabolism, as directed by genes, has to make a decision. Some of the homocysteine surely is needed to make cysteine and what comes from it (GSH, taurine, insulin, enzymes, body proteins and peptides). If there's inflammation going on, certain genes will be expressed to emphasize the route to cysteine, so that lots of GSH can be made. If this is the emphasis, then by default, there's less emphasis on adding to the stores of methionine and SAM for methylation.

One possible consequence of less methylation is rigidity of fatty acids adjacent to neuronal receptors that process sensory signals from the outside. Proper action by these receptors allows neuronal networks to pay attention to news from the environment. These receptors cannot act properly if the adjacent fatty acids are not methylated, for then they are too stiff and inflexible. Dopamine D4 receptors are of this type, and we are indebted to Professor Richard Deth (Northeastern University) for his pioneering studies of the autistic condition and of the relevance of fatty acid methylation. When methylation of the membrane fatty acids adjacent to dopamine D4 receptors becomes inadequate, loss of neuronal synchrony results. (This produces the same result we'd get if phosphocreatine and ATP can't deliver energy on time to neurons.)

Now that you've got the picture of what's going on with methylation, let's follow cobalamin on its journey to help methylate whatever homocysteine is needed to remake methionine. When we last considered Cbl, it had been released from a liposome and joined with glutathione to form GSCbl. Here, the now-oxidized glutathione has reduced cobalt to the +2 oxidation state. GSCbl travels to a big enzyme complex that's going to promote a methyl transfer process. What happens next is further reduction of the oxidation state of cobalt from +2 to +1; simultaneously, glutathione says goodbye and leaves. The big enzyme complex is "methionine synthase" and the part that reduces cobalt's oxidation state is called "methionine synthase reductase". Very quickly (it's hoped!), SAM shows up and methylates Cbl+1 to form MeCbl, methylcobalamin (cobalt's then back to +2). The MeCbl then transfers the methyl to the enzyme apparatus that holds homocysteine nearby, and homocysteine receives the methyl, transforming it into methionine. With the methyl gone, Cbl+1 remains and very quickly again (we hope) methylated folate (5'-methyltetrahydrofolate) shows up to remethylate it back to MeCbl. From then on, Cbl and folate work together to methylate homocysteine. Folate as MeTHF brings the methyl to Cbl; MeCbl gives it to the transfer apparatus that adds it to homocysteine.

For many with ASD, I think there are three things that can go wrong. (1) SAM is slow to methylate because of an adenosine excess, (2) Regardless of adenosine, oxidants are too abundant and quick, and Cbl+1 gets oxidized to Cbl+2. (3) The individual has a genetic variant of the enzyme that forms the methyl carrier, MeTHF and its supply is not dependable enough to cope with oxidant and adenosine influences. What happens then is callup of a new GSCbl from lysosomes and, hopefully, prompt SAM methylation to restart the process.

All of this is the reason behind Dr. James Neubrander's protocol for regular, subcutaneous injections of methylcobalamin. (See DAN! Conference Proceedings (ARI): Fall 2005 pages 29-31, Spring 2004 p.241-252, Spring 2003 p 103-118.) Unfortunately, there is a wide variance in perceived outcomes for this therapy, with significant benefit reports ranging from about 15% to above 90%. What do the parents say? According to ARI Pub 34/March 2009, 72% report improved behaviors, 22% no effect, 4% worsened behaviors, n=899. Wow!

What we're about here isn't injecting stuff – that's medicine and the procedure has to be directed by an MD. How about oral B_{12}, usually as cyanocobalamin but also available as oral MeCbl? The reported benefits have varied year to year when data were kept, with improved behavior running at 50 to 60% - not bad.

This covers one of the two coenzyme tasks that cobalamin handles. The other one occurs inside mitochondria and the metabolic steps of concern are –

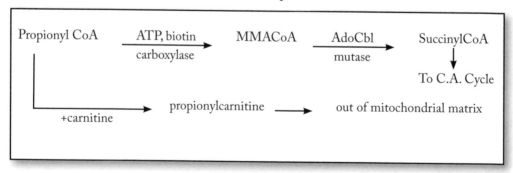

GSCbl passes through the mitochondrial membranes and meets a mitochondrial reductase enzyme that reduces Co+2 to Co+1. Oxidized glutathione leaves and has to be regenerated before it can again be useful. Right away, Cbl+1 meets a nearby adenosyl-transferase enzyme system that dumps the phosphates off ATP and connects adenosine to cobalamin.

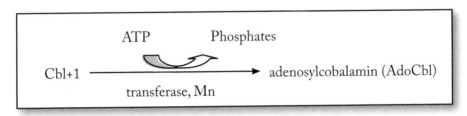

The transferase enzyme is a metal-activated flavoprotein that has riboflavin coenzyme as a part of its structure and manganese as an activator (Mn+2). And there's one more tech-nicality. Although this cobalt coenzyme is commonly called adenosylcobalamin, it's really made with a reduced adenosine, 5-deoxyadenosine. That's regular adenosine that's missing one oxygen atom on the ribose sugar part of the molecule.

What can go wrong with mitochondria coenzyme function of adenosylcobalamin? As with methylcobalamin, a glutathione shortage could limit the supply of usable GSCbl. Too much MMA from too much propionic acid can make it look like AdoCbl is deficient because this condition leads to elevated urine MMA – a telltale marker for vitamin B_{12} insufficiency. Deficient carnitine function can do exactly that because carnitine is supposed to remove propionate from the mitochondrial matrix. And carnitine formation requires three successive methylation of lysine by SAM. Reduced methylation with elevated ade-nosine (think inflammation) may lead to reduced carnitine levels. Then, if cyclosporins or other drugs come along and tie up the carnitine transporters, there will be an increased possibllity for mitochondrial dysfunction.

We don't see very many inborn errors of vitamin B_{12} metabolism in the autistic or ASD population, although I'm sure a few occur. Intrinsic factor and transcobalamin deficiencies occur but are relatively rare. Methionine synthase/reductase variants do occur and genetic testing can be done to identify these. We rarely see propionic academia, and the inborn errors for adenosylcobalamin formation are rare, too. What's not rare is mild-to-moderate elevations of urine MMA in about 25% of untreated children with ASD. So, something's wrong here and it's probably mitochondrial and related to the chemistry explained above.

Use of nitrous oxide, (N_2O) as an anesthetic disrupts B_{12} and folate metabolisms, and methionine synthase doesn't work as well as it should for three or four days afterward. Some dentists and anesthesiologists deny this; just about everybody else who has studied and published on the topic says it's so.

How Much Cobalamin Supplementation is Safe?

There's virtually no toxicity with regular cobalamin supplements, even at levels 1000x those that are government-suggested. You don't see urine cobalt increasing very much while cobalamin supplements are in use, because it's primarily excreted in bile/fecal matter. Also, whether it's methylcobalamin or cyanocobalamin or hydroxocobalamin, or the rarely used adenosylcobalamin, the cobalt is sequestered in the vitamin's chemical structure. Blood and cell levels of cobalt as measured by ICP-mass spectrometry will go up with cobalamin supplementation, because with such analytical procedures, the biochemical matrix of the blood cell specimen is totally destroyed prior to quantitative analysis. In the body, cobalt can't get out of the B_{12} structure.

Oral supplement levels of cyanocobalamin plus methylcobalamin may range from 20 to 1000 micrograms per serving (or per day). Personally, I doubt that amounts of less than 50 micrograms/day do much good for ASD individuals who need it.

About Folic Acid, Folate (Optional Reading)

The name folate comes from the Latin "folium" for leaf, and folic acid does come from leafy vegetables, such as spinach and parsley, but it also comes from meats, grains and beans. Many different types of yeast and some bacteria can synthesize it, too. In nature, folate exists with various amounts of attached glutamic acid. The vitamin is defined to be folate with just one attached glutamate – that's called folic acid or folacin, and it's not found that way in nature. Decades ago, the various glutamic acid attachments caused confusion about what the vitamin was. The triglutamate was 'fermentation factor", the heptaglutamate was a yeast-source type. It's been called vitamin Bc, Vitamin M, and anti-anemic factor. It wasn't until the 1940s that the chemistry and food sources of folic acid were well understood.

As with most vitamins, folate has to be processed in our tissues to be useful. All but one of the glutamates has to be removed (enzymatically), and then the resulting folic acid has to be activated. In this case, activation is chemical reduction by addition of lots of hydrogen – four atoms of hydrogen per molecule of folic acid. To make tetrahydrofolate, an active coenzyme/cofactor form of niacin is needed; either NADH or NADPH can be the hydrogen supplier. The resulting tetrahydrofolate is often abbreviated as THF.

Once formed, THF is a molecular truck that can acquire, carry and give away chemical parts that are composed of one carbon atom, some hydrogen, and maybe oxygen or nitrogen. These various parts are called "one carbon groups" by biochemists. I've listed some one-carbon groups below in the hope that name recognition will be helpful to you in learning more about what folic acid does in our bodies. The hyphens next to these one-carbon parts are carbon bonds, attachments that connect to neighboring atoms in THF or in molecules that get the carbon part from THF. All of these carbon parts are extremely important to human life and health.

$-CH_3$ is methyl
$=CH_2$ is methylene
$\equiv CH$ is methenyl
$-CHO$ is formyl
$-CH=NH$ is formimino

What does THF do with these various one-carbon parts?
- It carries methyls to cobalamin on methionine synthase enzymes to methylate homocysteine, remaking methionine. (See previous section, **About Cobalamin**.)
- THF provides methenyl and formyl parts to the purine assembly line in our cells where inosine is made. Insosine becomes adenosine and guanosine (for ATP and GTP), or adenine and guanine (for DNA). Without ATP, there's no adenosine to make SAM.
- THF provides methylene to the pyrimidine assembly line so that thymidine can be made from uridine. Sorry for the big words, but when this doesn't happen,

a possible consequence is "Fragile X Syndrome", which can feature autism and mental retardation. This disaster can happen during fetal development, and reversing it after birth with folate supplements doesn't work. However, ongoing problems due to continuing dietary folate inadequacy, such as poor methylation, can be corrected.

The funny-sounding one carbon part, formimino, is made when the THF meets up with a substance that comes from the dietary amino acid histidine. That substance has a long chemistry name, and since we've had enough of that already, let's use its abbreviation, FIGlu. (The Glu part stands for glutamic acid.)

My experience is that for ASD, it's unusual to normalize a high FIGlu condition by just giving a folate supplement. Often, methylcobalamin, TMG or DMG, antioxidants or even L-carnitine provide more help. Also, when a folate supplement does help, it's more likely to be folinic acid than either folic acid or methylTHF. MethylTHF has to give its methyl away before it can do anything else, and the major give-away site is cobalamin on methionine synthase. If that's malfunctioning then THF is trapped as methylTHF. Folinic acid is the THF carrying the formyl part (-CHO). Folinic acid exchanges well with other THF forms and is less likely to wind up stuck at methionine synthase.

There's one instance in ASD where supplemental methylTHF could be specifically helpful. That's when there's a genetic variant with weakness in the enzyme (MTHFR) that makes methylTHF. MTHFR weakness can be identified by a genetic test that your doctor can order. Be advised, you're not guaranteed a problem-fix by supplementing methylTHF when the test does show MTHFR weakness. Problems upstream in the biochemistry in ASD seem to be the case in at least two out of three with variant MTHFR. Upstream problems include adenosine excess, glutathione insufficiency, and cobalamin supply problems. (With today's knowledge of this subject, do <u>not</u> rely on genetics testing to tell you what's wrong. So far in ASD, this just hasn't been productive.)

Other than the possible folate trap problem, what other situations are there that increase need for folic acid and use of folic acid/folinic acid supplements?

- Maldigestion/malabsorption syndromes
- Junk food diet
- Oxidant stress or chemical toxicity that impairs folic acid activation by NADH/NADPH
- Use of medications that are folate antagonists: nonsteroidal antiinflammatories (NSAIDS), methyltrexate, cholestyramine, valproate, colchicines, sulfasalazine, phenytoin, phenobarbital. Health professionals should be able to help with this.
- Consumption of alcoholic beverages or intestinal yeast overgrowth with autobrewery syndrome.

From my experience, a multivitamin containing 400 micrograms/serving (per day) of folate as folinic acid or folinic + folic acids does the job for children aged 5 and above. Cut it in half for 2 year olds. Try 5-methylTHF (FolaPro™) only when you have evidence of a MTHFR problem because you might otherwise make things worse. The multivitamin you're using should contain vitamin B$_{12}$ when it contains folate. Do not supplement folic acid as a stand-alone vitamin unless you also supplement vitamin B$_{12}$.

Comment – Every so often, a well-meaning medical authority, usually an academic, decides to blame autism on excesses of dietary folate, particularly the amount that's added to "fortify" processed foods, plus dietary supplements. They've "discovered" that methylation, one-carbon chemistry, etc. could have something to do with autism! Well, folate in food or supplements does not cause autism. But autism can and does, to some extent, feature folate metabolism problems such as methylTHF traps and the mysterious and probably complicated FIGlu dilemma.

Vitamin A and Beta-Carotene

Vitamin A was named retinol in recognition of its essential role in the chemistry of vision. Vitamin A also is a slight exception to vitamins not being part of body structure. The pigment, rhodopsin (visual purple) in the retina of the eye is a protein combined with vitamin A. When light strikes rhodopsin, it splits into two parts, the protein piece (opsin) and retinene, also called vitamin A aldehyde or "retinal". Retinol or vitamin A (by definition) is an alcohol form. When rhodopsin is split and retinal is formed, several colored substances also are produced. Retinal is in all of the generated colors; the difference in the colors is due to differences in the protein or opsin parts.

In animal-source foods (meat, fish, fowl), vitamin A exists primarily as retinol. In vegetable foods, vitamin A exists as beta-carotene – especially in yellow or orange-colored ones. Beta-carotene is similar to two retinals stuck together. Sometimes called pro-vitamin A, beta-carotene is more stable and more enduring than retinal or retinol. Vitamin A as retinal is produced enzymatically in the liver from beta-carotene by splitting it in two and adding oxygen to each piece. Typically, this isn't a very efficient conversion, and humans need quite a bit of beta-carotene to form the required amount of vitamin A.

Indications of Need

All of the following are consistent with increased need for vitamin A: difficulty with visual acuity in dim light, dryness and/or thickening of ocular tissues, thickening and hardening of the skin (hyperkeratosis), loss of skin hair due to obstructed follicles, frequent infections, nasal or intestinal mucus deficiency, immunodeficiency (reduced T-lymphocyte cell function), and oxidant stress and inflammation, A blood vitamin analysis might have results indicating vitamin A and/or beta-carotene insufficiency. Protein malnutrition and diet of carbohydrates lacking sufficient beta-carotene can also result in deficiency of this vitamin. With ASD, we're particularly concerned about vitamin A's help in decreasing the incidence of infection and inflammation.

When and How Much

Vitamin A alone, as cod liver oil, or in multivitamin products can be given at the beginning stage of nutritional intervention. Breakfast, dinner, or bedtime servings make little difference in my experience. The how much part is more complicated because of rather confusing aspects of vitamin A measurement units. In older literature on vitamins you will find vitamin A measured only in International Units (IU). 1.0 IU of vitamin A is 0.30 micrograms of all-trans-retinol, and 1.0 IU of vitamin A as beta-carotene is (was) equivalent to 0.60 micrograms of beta-carotene. This has been superseded by new units of measurement and new recommendations. The units in current use are retinol equivalents (RE). 1.0 RE is the same as 3.33 IU of vitamin A. 1.0 RE = 1.0 microgram of all trans-retinol = 6.0 micrograms of all trans-beta-carotene. "All Trans" refers to the configuration of some of the carbon-to-carbon bonds in the molecules – something that's taken into account during vitamin A supplement manufacture and accounted for by the product label. The equivalent amount of beta-carotene is higher because of estimated inefficiencies in dietary uptake and conversion to retinol. Multivitamin products providing vitamin A also should contain beta-carotene which has important antioxidant functions on its own (see also vitamin E section).

The current Food and Nutrition Board (Institute of Medicine) recommended amounts for vitamin A, stated in RE or micrograms (they are the same) or IU are –

AGE/CONDITION	VITAMIN A (RE) or mcg	IU(approx)
Birth-6 months	375	1250
6 months – 1 year	375	1250
1-3 years	400	1330
4-6 years	500	1660
7-10 years	700	2330
Females 11 yrs and older	800	2660
Pregnant female	800	2660
Lactating female	1300 (first 6 mos)	4330
Lactating female	1200 (second 6 mos)	4000
Males 11 and older	1000	3330

Remember that I said that FDA regulations for product labeling are different from what the Food and Nutrition Board recommends? Well, the FDA Daily Value or "serving" is the same as it has been for decades for vitamin A, 5000 IU. That is an adult amount or an amount that corresponds to a 2000 calorie/day diet. If your supplement bottle says 4000 IU of vitamin A per serving, then you've got 80% of the FDA's reference amount for daily intake.

What about the problem that vitamin A is an oil (a liquid) but the vitamin bottle contains capsules or tablets? This, of course, is not a problem for fish oil supplements like cod liver oil. That's natural vitamin A. But for packaging in capsules or tablets, manufacturers need solids in powder form. What is most often used is a synthetic esterified form, retinyl acetate. You need about 15% more retinyl acetate to equal a given amount of vitamin A. About 1150 RE of retinyl acetate provides the same activity as 1000 RE of all-trans-retinol. There is a way to provide natural retinol that's solid-like for capsule formulations, using spray-absorption onto carrier particles, but this is expensive and unusual.

If you're using beta-carotene to provide vitamin A activity, you need to know three things. First, beta-carotene is stored and converted to vitamin A at your liver's convenience. Human infants and some young children don't make this conversion efficiently. In some, the conversion is extremely limited. It isn't possible to produce hypervitaminosis A by taking large doses of beta-carotene. But if large amounts are used, the skin may turn reddish-brown from lots of stored beta-carotene. Second, if you have pure, all trans-beta carotene, then to get 1000 RE you typically need about 6000 micrograms of that type of beta-carotene. Third, with other carotenes, even more is needed. If you have a natural blend of provitamin A carotenoids, from some plant source, then to get 1000 RE you need 12,000 micrograms of the mixed carotenoids.

Medical warnings about excessive use of vitamin A during pregnancy stem from the possibility of birth defects which have been rare in humans, but have occurred more frequently in animal tests of high-dose vitamin A. Actual vitamin A toxicity from hypervitaminosis A is rare. But you can get into trouble with really excessive amounts. The pharmacy handbook Drug Facts and Comparisons lists the following levels (excluding pregnancy) that correspond to acute toxicity (single dose) –

> Infants less than 1 year old, 100,000 IU/dose
> Children 1 to 6 years old, 100,000 IU/dose
> Adults, 1,000,000 IU/dose
>
> For chronic toxicity –
> Infants, 18,500 IU/day for one to three months
> Adults, 50,000 IU/day for longer than 18 months
> or 500,000 IU/day for two months.

My suggestions for vitamin A supplementation for ASD are –
1. Don't forget to supplement taurine
2. Use a multivitamin that provides 3000 to 5000 IU via a mixture of retinal (30-60%) and beta-carotene (60-30%) for children 5 years old and older. Cut this in half for 3-5 year olds. See your doctor or nutrition counselor for those younger than three years.
3. If there is evidence of special need for more vitamin A or more is professionally recommended, provide some or all of the additional amounts as cod liver oil (contains vitamins A and D). Ensure that your cod liver oil is certified by the manufacturer or purified to remove mercury and heavy elements and other possible toxicants.

Adverse Responses to Vitamin A

According to the ARI Parent Response Tally for supplements (ARI Publ. 34, March 2009), only 3% of 1535 responses, or 46 instances of worse behavior, have been reported from the ASD population. The simplest solution to a bad response is to discontinue the supplement. Unfortunately, the biological half-life of vitamin A in humans is 3 to 6 weeks (because it's an oil), so symptoms may be slow to disappear. This is a good reason for starting with low supplement amounts. Quantity, purity or metabolism could be behind an adverse response.

Symptoms of hypervitaminosis A include –

Headache, dizziness, nausea, weakness, muscle stiffness, joint or bone pain, loss of hair for chronic overdosing, and sometimes a skin rash, often at the back of the neck.

Is taurine insufficient? Taurine helps to detoxify used vitamin A.

Vitamin A has several natural forms including retinyl palmitate, which is in fish liver oils. Palmitate or palmitic acid is a natural long-chain oil that naturally exists in many animals and vegetables. A very small subset of humans seems to have allergic-like sensitivity to palmitate, and this may actually be "cross-reactivity" to something else. Food allergies usually involve proteins or peptides, not fatty acids. Yet respected allergists, such as Theron Randolph MD (now deceased), reported sensitivity to palm oil and palmitate. So, one possible remedy is to switch to another type of vitamin A, perhaps to vitamin A acetate, even though it is a synthetic form. If a child shows reactivity to coconut on a food allergy test and has trouble with vitamin A palmitate, then you have a good reason to try another type of vitamin A.

About Vitamin A (Optional Reading)

Vitamin A is called the "anti-infective vitamin". Pharmacologically, it is defined to be one molecular structure, "all-trans-retinol". In nature (animals, not plants) there are several vitamin A-like molecules having vitamin A activities of various degrees. Fish oils, especially cod liver oil, contain several vitamin A forms, predominantly the esterified retinyl palmitate form. Esterified means that it's attached to another molecule which often increases the stability of the vitamin. Fish oils also contain some vitamin D. While plants do not contain vitamins A or D, they do contain a precursor for vitamin A, provitamin A or beta-carotene. Vitamin A is of interest in autism because it seems to improve immune function, has protective actions for cell mitochondria, and because it may not be well absorbed from food sources when there's intestinal disorder.

In 1999, Mary Megson, MD postulated that vitamin A can help alleviate defective G-alpha protein function in autism [*Med Hypotheses* 54 (2000) 979-83]. The G-alpha protein is part of a cell's signal transmission system located in the outer (plasma) membrane of the neuron. It gives signal transmission an energy push by releasing phosphate from GTP to form GDP. This chemical change provides energy to some of the chemistry that moves a message from the cell membrane receptor into the cell's inner workings. Dr. Megson did this research with patients who had family histories of G-alpha protein defect. DAN! studies and studies by others of autistic populations have not confirmed defective G-alpha protein as a commonality in ASD. However, there is very strong circumstantial evidence for GTP energy supply deficit in brain cells in autism. Included in this evidence are the findings of low brain ATP and phosphocreatine by Minshew et al, *Biol Psych* 33 (1993) 762-73. Whether or not vitamin A supplements help cellular perception when brain ATP or phosphocreatine are insufficient is not known. There are numerous anecdotal reports of improvement with supplementation of nutritional amounts of natural vitamin A (as in cod liver oil.)

Use of vitamin A has been proposed to combat entrenched viral infections, those that seem static and unaffected (or at least unconquered) by the autistic person's immune system. This use of vitamin A is controversial. Antiviral use involves megadose amounts of vitamin A, up to 100,000 IU/day (30,000 RE/day) for short periods (days). Presentations by doctors at autism conferences have not described incidents of hypervitaminosis A in older children or adults with these amounts. Neither do they report any consensus about viral cures or normalization of viral titers including measles. While there are anecdotal reports of significant improvement, most do not show such responses with megadose A. Therapeutic dosing of children with vitamin A should be done only under the direction of a physician.

Recent publications in medical and scientific literature support the contention that vitamin A depletion can lead to immunodeficiency, oxidant stress and mitochondrial dysfunction. The immunodeficiency can result from death of T-lymphocyte cells; oxidant stress from generation of reactive oxygen species ("ROS"), and mitochondrial dysfunction from membrane damage. Chiu HJ, Fischman DA, Hammerling U, *FASEB Journal* 2008 Nov, 22 (11) 3878-87.

Lymphocyte differentiation – selection and development of T and B cells for proper immune response is regulated, in part, by vitamin A – Manicassarny A and Pulendran B, *Semin.Immunol* 2009 Feb, 21 (1) 22-27.

Secretion of immunoglobulin A (IgA) by mucosal cells in the intestines depends, in part, on vitamin A – More JR, Iwata M et al. *Science* 2006 Nov. 314 (5802) 1157-60.

Vitamin A supplementation enhances immunoglobulin production and downregulates inflammatory responses – Aukrust P, Müller F et al. *Eur J. Clin Invest*, 2000 Mar, 30(3) 252-59

Vitamin C

Besides its commonly recognized benefits of antioxidant activity and alleviating constipation, vitamin C has several biological functions that can be very important in ASD, including its role in carnitine synthesis.

Based on over 3000 parent responses to ARI about benefits to behavior vs worsening, vitamin C gets a "gold star"! Over 1400 "got better" (46%) while only about 65 "got worse" (2%). That better/worse ratio exceeds 20!

Indications of Need

Symptoms consistent with need for vitamin C include: constipation, inflamed or bleeding gums, rough/inflamed patches or papules on skin (hyperkeratosis), petechiae, hemorrhagic skin spots, frequent/constant signs of inflammation, general weakness, lack of physical endurance and frequent infections. Laboratory test results consistent with oxidant stress or iron deficiency are also indicative. Dietary ascorbate enhances the uptake of dietary iron.

When and How Much?

For autistic children weighing less than about 50 lbs (23 Kg), about 250 mg/d is the usually suggested amount, and that is the initial trial dose as well. For children at 50 to 100 lb, 500 mg/d or more (per physician's direction) can be used. Usually, 500 to 1000 mg/d is the minimum that is adequate for autistic individuals weighing over 100 lbs. I usually do not suggest use of more than 2000 mg/d except for short periods of time, such as may be needed to counteract constipation. From my experience, breakfast and/or lunch are the best times for vitamin C supplements. Use with supper may lead to multiple potty trips at night. Give stand-alone vitamin C supplements at different times/meals from vitamin B_{12} supplements.

Adverse Responses to Vitamin C?

As summarized above, adverse responses are uncommon. Most have been excessively loose stools or diarrhea. Often, this is due to too much of the laxative-acting supplements: magnesium, citrates, phosphatidylcholine, herbals, as well as vitamin C.

Occasionally, individuals with extreme sensitivity (allergy) to corn will have trouble with vitamin C supplements. Non-corn-based vitamin C is available – check with a nutritionist or call suppliers. Most health food stores carry brands that are corn-based vitamin C; the non-corn based ascorbate does cost more. 99.9% pure, hypoallergenic vitamin C has very few reports of allergy problems.

Multi-element buffered vitamin C may be the answer when amounts over 500 mg/d are to be used. Bowel tolerance is much better for this type of ascorbate. Also, multi-element buffered C replenishes elements (calcium, magnesium, potassium, etc.) that can be lost in urine when ascorbic acid is supplemented.

About Vitamin C (Optional Reading)

Vitamin C's chemical name is ascorbic acid, and it can be combined with elements (minerals) to make salt forms such as calcium ascorbate, magnesium ascorbate, potassium ascorbate, etc. When these salt forms are manufactured, the acidic property of vitamin C is counteracted. Blends of ascorbic acid and ascorbate salts can then be formulated such that mild acidity, neutrality, or mild alkalinity results. In other words, ascorbate supplements can be custom-made so as to not upset even delicate acid-base balances.

Many mammals can synthesize their own vitamin C from dietary sugar or glucose. Ascorbate is not really a vitamin for them; it's a natural biochemical that they make internally. Cats and dogs can make anywhere from 5 to 40 mg of vitamin C per day per kilogram of body weight. Animals that aren't very careful about their eating habits can make much more (and need it) – goats 32 to 190 and rats 40 to 200 mg/kg of body weight per day. The same authoritative reference that states these amounts (*New England Journal of Medicine*, April 3, 1986) also states the US government-established recommended dietary allowance for humans in the same units of measurement, 0.9 mg/kg per day. Humans cannot form vitamin C because we lack one of the required enzymes. So, for us, ascorbate is a vitamin. It looks like we've been shortchanged here, doesn't it? Actually, the Food and Nutrition Board of the National Research Council did make some minor progress on this issue. In the 1970s the adult RDA for vitamin C was 45 mg/day. In the late 1980s it became 60 mg/day, a 33% increase. Looking at the pharmacy handbook, Facts and Comparisons (January 2003 update page), the RDA or DRI still is 60 mg but the experts are beginning to hedge upward for those with special needs. If you use nicotine (smoke or chew tobacco), you should take at least 100 mg/d. "The average protective dose is 70 to 150 mg/day" (for adults, "protection" is not explained). For scurvy, 300 to 1000 mg/day is stated. For enhanced wound healing, 300 to 500 mg/d for 7 to 10 days, and for severe burns, 1000 to 2000 mg/d is suggested. Also mentioned in this edition of Facts and Comparisons is: "… up to 6 grams per day has been administered intravenously to healthy adults without evidence of toxicity." But there are warnings for diabetics and those with recurrent kidney stones. For those individuals, high-dose vitamin C might be detrimental.

What exactly does vitamin C do in the human body? And why would it be beneficial in autism?

1. Antioxidant functions. Certain cells in the blood carry out a protective role when they meet up with stuff that doesn't belong. Neutrophils can do this, and they are able to use several methods to dispatch what's unwanted. The unwanted stuff includes various microbes, certain types of viruses, toxic agents, and even very fine particles, such as might come from engine exhaust that is inhaled and absorbed from the lungs. Enzymatic digestion, chemical oxidation and other destructive means can be used by these phagocytic cells. The oxidation activity is of concern in ASD because of all the findings of oxidant stress and oxidant damage. Vitamin C neutralizes reactive types of oxygen and hydroxide, and is seen as protective against oxidant stress that might occur with infectious toxins, or toxicant chemical exposures.

2. Assembly of carnitine. Inside most of our cells are little compartments that do chemical energy generation as well as other crucial tasks. Called mitochondria, they need fuel for their energy generation processes, and a lot of that fuel comes from dietary fats. But getting fats (fatty acids), or anything else, into a mitochondrion, isn't going to happen without a passport and an escort. Carnitine is a big-time escort with a passport (it's accepted at special ports of entry), and it carries fatty acids through the inner mitochondrial membrane. (See chapter on carnitine.) The final enzymatic step in carnitine's assembly process uses vitamin C as a promoter. Because mitochondrial process including carnitine's functions have been discovered to be issues of concern in ASD, we have good reason to be concerned about vitamin C adequacy.

3. Potentiation of oxytocin. Oxytocin is a peptide with important hormonal functions. Peptides are chains of amino acids that body organs or tissues assemble; oxytocin is made in the brain (hypothalamus) where it is transported to nerves in the posterior pituitary where it is released into blood circulation. It also is used in the brain where it influences social interaction. In clinical studies, giving oxytocin has improved social engagement for autistics. For Mom after birth, oxytocin promotes milk ejection from mammary glands. Oxytocin levels, oxytocin-forming genes and oxytocin receptors all are under study for their possible roles in ASD.
In 1986, Mark Levine, MD, authored a review article on ascorbate for the *New England Journal of Medicine* (April 3, vol. 314, issue no.4, p 892-902). In that authoritative review, Dr. Levine cited four research publications that deal with the chemistry of peptide hormones with explicit mention of oxytocin. An enzyme that "mediates" (influences) oxytocin formation is thought to have "maximal activity" when ascorbate assists as a reducing agent - another possible benefit of vitamin C for ASD.

4. Formation of folinic acid. Studies of metabolism in ASD populations have often concluded that, for some, the biochemistry of folic acid is messed up or clogged up. This may be of genetic origin, or due to toxicant exposure, or for reasons we don't know yet. Regardless, one potential problem is that of adding hydrogen atoms to the vitamin known as folic acid or folate. One active form is tetrahydrofolate (THF), having four added hydrogens. Another active form is folinic acid. Folinic

acid also has four added hydrogen atoms, but some are in places on the molecule that differ from tetrahydrofolate. Folinic acid also carries a carbon (formyl) group that adds to its usefulness and versatility. It is vitamin C that potentiates the addition of the active carbon group on folinic acid (Drug Facts & Comparisons, Jan 2003 p 19; Harper et al. Review of Physiological Chemistry 17th Ed, 1979, p 172). Folinic acid can feed into folate metabolism in places where tetrahydrofolate cannot and also where methyl tetrahydrofolate cannot.

5. Metabolic assist for catecholamines and phenylalanine/tyrosine. Catecholamines are a class of neurotransmitters, and we've all heard of some of them – dopamine, adrenaline (epinephrine), norepinephrine, etc. Much of the essential amino acid phenylalanine becomes tyrosine, another amino acid, and tyrosine is the starting material for catecholamine synthesis. It's also the basis of thyroid hormone. But only a little bit of tyrosine is used for these purposes. A lot of it goes into protein formation for body tissues. Tyrosine that's left over goes through an oxidation/catabolism sequence that contributes to the supply of acetyl-coenzyme A. Acetyl-CoA is fuel for the energy conversion process (citric acid cycle) in cell mitochondria. There are vitamin C-potentiated steps in two branches of tyrosine metabolism – the catecholamine branch and the oxidative catabolism branch. This is biochemistry that must work efficiently, especially when trying to improve the autistic condition.

6. Cleanup assist for antipsychotic medications. For a number of years, our son required haloperidol ("Haldol") to control his behavior. This was before we were able to control his diet with the exclusion of casein. Nothing else worked. We desired use of the minimum Haldol dose that did the job of alleviating aggressive, destructive behaviors. We were able to do this with 0.1 mg doses twice a day whereas the doctors had started with 0.5 mg three times per day and were expecting to have to increase it. He was also getting 1000 mg/d ascorbate. We did not know how this was possible, but the 0.1 mg doses worked. In 1985, the answer appeared in Science Magazine. Ascorbate potentiates Haldol and some other antipsychotics, probably by prolonging the biologic effect of the medication in the body by clearing the neuronal receptor sites where it binds to elicit its antipsychotic effect. See Literature-Vitamins, Rebec, G, Centors J et al. cited at the end of the chapter.

Correcting some misperceptions about vitamin C

Vitamin C is not a chelating agent; it doesn't chelate anything. Ascorbic acid might form a compound (salt) with a toxicant element, like lead, and be excreted as lead ascorbate. This is pure hypothesis as far as I know, but still, that's not chelation.

Vitamin C, at the supplement amounts described here, is very unlikely to form oxalate in the body. Studies done years ago showed that oxalate formed in the urine specimens of individuals who took multi-gram amounts of ascorbic acid. This was attributed to oxidation in the aging urine before it was analyzed. Prompt (immediate) analysis of urine from the same individuals showed negligible oxalate. If you want a medical textbook statement on this, see Hillman R "Primary Hyperoxalurias", Chapter 25 in Scriver et al., Eds, The Metabolic Basis of Inherited Disease, 6th ed, McGraw-Hill (1989) page 935 and 938 – less than 4 grams/day ascorbate intake does not increase urinary oxalate (adults).

"Vitamin C destroys vitamin B_{12}". This is bunk that originated with laboratory bench studies of putting B_{12} into a flask containing dissolved ascorbic acid. This does not reflect what happens in real life. It is, however, advisable to separate stand-alone oral vitamin B_{12} supplements, such as methylcobalamin, from stand-alone ascorbate or ascorbic acid supplements – give them at different meals.

Vitamin D

For many years, vitamin D has been recognized only for its role in regulating calcium metabolism. In fact, we're now learning that it does a whole lot more including enhancment of our primary antioxidant cofactor, NADPH. Additionally, vitamin D activates a protein that functions to rebalance biochemical reduction-oxidation (redox) processes in cells. Normally, it is nutritionally essential only when we're not exposed to adequate sunlight (face, hands and arms for about 20 minutes per day). With adequate sunlight (the ultraviolet part) and with normal physiology, we make enough vitamin D from cholesterol in our own tissues. However, even with sunlight, there can be a vitamin D adequacy problem when there's persistent oxidant stress or when cells are out of balance in their redox regulation capabilities, as with malignancy. With ASD we're often concerned with overcoming oxidant stress due to limitations in NADPH and GSH.

Indications of Need

These include: laboratory test results or symptoms consistent with oxidant stress, or low GSH (reduced glutathione) per analysis. Subnormal vitamin D per blood analysis is a definite indicator of need. Limited daily exposure to direct sunlight is another, as are intestinal malabsorption or increased fat content of stools. Insomnia, nervousness and irritation/burning sensation in the mouth and/or throat have been reported in some cases of vitamin D deficiency. Every person with autism/ASD should get a supplemental vitamin D in an amount at least equal to the recommended quantities (servings) for their age.

When and How Much?

As part of a daily vitamin regimen, those with ASD would be expected to benefit from: 50 to 100 IU/d for age 1 to 2 years; 100 to 200 IU/d for age 3-10 years; 200 to 400 IU/d for age 11 and above. Vitamin D quantities are in USP units or IU units traditionally, and the FDA (adult) daily serving amount is 400 IU. One (1) IU is 0.025 micrograms, either for vitamin D_2 (ergocalciferol) or D_3 (cholecalciferol). 400 IU is 10 micrograms of vitamin D.

A vitamin D analysis (blood) is advisable, except that a "normal" blood level may not actually be adequate when oxidant stress with inflammation is a persistent condition. The value of such a test is in finding subnormal levels. In my experience, hypervitaminosis D is rare and I've not gotten reports of it with children (age 3 to 10 years) taking the adult serving amounts (400 IU/d), nor have I heard of adults having problems with three times that (1200 IU/d). For supplemental amounts above this, have a good reason and have medical supervision. You can start vitamin D supplements when you begin the vitamin trials during Tier 1 of the supplement intervention schedule. Use the D_3, cholecalciferol, form. If you are using a vitamin D supplement that is separate from a multivitamin, then the supper meal (when calcium is given) is a good time for the vitamin D capsule.

Adverse Response to Vitamin D?

The only reports to me about problems with appropriate levels of supplemental vitamin D have occurred for people with poor kidney function or who, for some reason, have elevated blood calcium levels. Increased blood creatinine with apparently normal kidney function is a warning condition and a contraindication for vitamin D supplementation, but this is rare in ASD. Symptoms consistent with vitamin D excess include dry mouth and thirst, metallic taste, loss of appetite, nausea, headache, and general weakness.

If, by mistake, a large amount (several capsules) of vitamin D is swallowed, then prompt mineral oil by mouth will increase fecal excretion; later give lots of water to drink.

About Vitamin D (Optional Reading)

First of all, it's a stretch to call this stuff a vitamin. It's a hormone that is made from cholesterol, the source of some of our other hormones. What's different about vitamin D is that the really active form requires an ultraviolet energy input during its assembly.

Vitamin D_1, by definition, is a blend of vitamin D_2 and lumisterol. Lumisterol is a chemical cousin of cholesterol. Now that you know this, you can forget it; D_1 is a lousy form of supplemental vitamin D.

Vitamin D_2 is called calciferol or ergocalciferol or oleovitamin D_2, and it has lots of other commercial names. D_2 is made naturally in plants by photolysis. It's not much good either because UV light (sunlight) still is needed to progress to the active form of D.

Vitamin D_3 is called cholecalciferol or oleovitamin D_3 or "activated" 7-dehydrocholesterol (cholesterol without one of its hydrogen atoms). While it's called "activated", it's not really the active form of the vitamin – it's just one important step closer than was D_2. D_3 is what our bodies make using UV energy in sunlight to knock off one hydrogen atom. This occurs, of course, in skin. The reason D_3 is a good supplement form is because it's the dehydrogenated form, and no more sunshine is needed to get to the active forms.

The D_3 in food or the D_3 made in our skin next goes to the liver. There, the carbon atom number 25 on D_3 gets a hydroxyl group (-OH, oxygen and hydrogen) added to it. The result is 25-hydroxycholecalciferol; it's an intermediate or storage form of vitamin D.

Finally, one of two possible final activation steps occurs to our 25-hydroxy D_3. In kidney, bone and placental tissue, the number 1 carbon also gets an –OH attached to make 1,25-dihydroxyD_3. This is the most potent hormonal form of the vitamin. It and parathyroid hormones control calcium metabolism.

A second form made in the same tissues plus the intestines is 24,25 dihydroxy D_3. It acts as a throttle or balancer to the 1,25-dihydroxy D_3 form, and it influences uptake of dietary calcium.

Okay, this probably is more than you ever wanted to know about how our bodies make vitamin D, but now you've got the whole picture – except what vitamin D does that might benefit the autistic condition. There are three biochemical benefits that vitamin D might provide.

First, 1,25-dihydroxy D_3 can enhance the genetic mechanism for formation of the enzyme glucose-6-phosphate dehydrogenase or G6PD. This is the enzyme that puts hydrogen on NADP to make our top-grade antioxidant cofactor NADPH (go back and read the niacin part of the B-vitamin chapter if you don't remember NADPH). We need NADPH to recycle oxidized glutathione and get back the active GSH form.

Second, 1,25 dihydroxy D_3 can enhance the genetic mechanism for formation of the enzyme cystathionine beta-synthase. That enzyme processes homocysteine into cystathionine, cystathionine then forms cysteine, and cysteine is needed to make glutathione or taurine or sulfate or metallothionein or oxytocin or G6PD or any of the other many cysteine-containing biochemicals in our bodies.

Third, both forms of dihydroxy D_3, working together, modulate calcium binding/transporting proteins including proteins that hold calcium in neurons and interneurons. In interneurons, calcium binding often has GABA as a neighbor. Some neuronal structures in brain tissue that incorporate calcium binding sites develop as the brain develops and as network synchrony becomes necessary for perception and response to external news. Without adequate calcium binding, some of this synchrony won't occur. So, adequate vitamin D is really essential for the brain to develop properly. Remember also that one of taurine's functions is to look after neuronal calcium levels – teamwork is what nutrients are all about.

Scientific studies published in the last decade also indicate that activated vitamin D has immunomodulation and anti-inflammatory functions such as down-regulation of inflammatory cytokines. We're still learning about his hormone's complex but profound contributions to human development and health.

Vitamin E

As with vitamins A, C, and D, vitamin E is available as a stand-alone supplement and as an ingredient in multivitamin formulations. We're interested in supplemental vitamin E for those with autism and ASD because of its antioxidant and tissue-protective properties.

Indications of Need

Supplemental vitamin E may be beneficial when there are laboratory test results consistent with oxidant stress/damage and/or inflammation, or low blood plasma/serum tocopherol levels (<0.5 mg/dl). Those with intestinal malabsorption, especially fat malabsorption (excess stool fat), taurine or biliary insufficiency, or clay-colored stools are likely to be deficient in vitamin E. Premature infants and those with any form of gastrointestinal distress also are prone to this deficiency. Symptoms of inadequate vitamin E are diverse and may not be apparent. Chronic or episodic inflammation, easy bruising with breakage of red blood cells (hemolysis), muscle aches/weakness, dull hair, falling hair, and neuromuscular disorders are additional possible indications of need for vitamin E. Limited glutathione stores (by laboratory assay) is a definite indicator of need.

When and How Much?

If it's included in the daily multivitamin (a Tier 1 supplement), that's fine. If your nutritionist or doctor suggests an additional amount, then I'd opt for supper time for the stand-alone vitamin E. In my experience, additional stand-alone vitamin E supplementation often is beneficial.

There are a half dozen different chemical forms (tocopherols) that make up the vitamin E family, but the 'alpha"-tocopherol form is defined to be the vitamin for unit potency purposes. Even that doesn't make things simple because there are: synthetic (solid) d,l-alpha-tocopherol acetate, natural liquid d-alpha-tocopherol and natural solidified d-alpha-tocopherol acetate. Adding acetate makes natural and synthetic tocopherols into solids or powders, whereas without acetate they are oily liquids.

For synthetic, solid, d,l-α-tocopherol acetate, 1.0 mg = 1.0 IU (often purer, easy to package, least potency)

For natural, solid d-α-tocopherol acetate, 1.0 mg = 1.36 IU (easy to package)

For natural, liquid d-α-tocopherol, 1.0 mg = 1.49 IU (highest potency)

The Food and Nutrition Board of the NRC (now under the Institute of Medicine, IOM) listed very small RDA levels of vitamin E (d-α-tocopherol) for children, about 4 to 10 milligrams per day (10th Ed RDA, NRC, National Academy Press, 1989). For many with ASD, these small amounts won't be adequate. I recommend the following supplement ranges for d-α-tocopherol. If tolerated, you may try a "natural" product that includes additional tocopherols (see below). Natural mixed tocopherol supplements are oils usually refined from corn oil. Higher amounts may be beneficial, but seek medical direction before doing that.

Age (years)	IU/day
1-3	15-30
4-6	25-50
7-10	40-80
Males 11-14	50-100
Males 15-18	60-120
Females 11-14	45-90
Females 15-18	50-100

Adverse Response to Vitamin E?

If you are using natural vitamin E, most likely it is corn-based. Rarely, exquisite corn-reactors can develop an adverse response with daily use of this form of vitamin E. This is quite uncommon; much less common than with corn-based vitamin C to which cornstarch is often added. Another concern, occasionally, with corn-based vitamin E is carryover of systemic crop sprays. I suggest changing brands before giving up on supplemental amounts of this nutrient. You'd have to use very large amounts of vitamin E to create a hypervitaminosis E toxicity condition – over 500 to 1000 IU/d in children and over 2000 to 3000 IU/d in adults. Somewhere in between proper levels and excessive megadoses, problems with slowed blood clotting can occur. Symptoms of excessive tocopherol levels include flatulence, nausea, headache, diarrhea, cramps, nosebleeds and muscle weakness. Too much vitamin E may also cause elevated cholesterol, elevated triglycerides and decreased thyroid hormone levels.

About Vitamin E (Optional Reading)

There are six naturally-occurring tocopherols, and they are distinguished by chemical structure, specifically by where methyls occur on the molecule. Each tocopherol is a vitamin E member of the total, natural vitamin E family. Each has slightly different activities or potencies for the various functions that the vitamin family attends to. The natural tocopherols are –

Alpha	5,7,8-trimethyl
Beta	5,8 dimethyl
Gamma	7,8-dimethyl
Delta	8-methyl
Eta	7-methyl
Zeta	5,7-dimethyl

Foods that contain vitamin E are plants, not animals or fish, and each kind of plant typically produces different amounts of all or most of these tocopherols. Such foods are: soybeans and soy oil, corn, safflower, wheat germ, sunflower seeds, olives, walnuts, sesame and peanuts. Vitamin E is a common food additive, used to retard oxidation of the food product. In this use, vitamin E is oxidized (sacrificed) in order to preserve the food itself.

The primary function of vitamin E is as an antioxidant in tissue that's exposed to moderate concentrations of oxygen or oxidants. Vitamin E defends against oxidation of lipid (fatty acid) membranes and peroxidation of phospholipids. For example, it helps protect lipids in neuronal membranes where the lipids are adjacent to receptor structures – like the attention-getting dopamine D4 receptor. Peroxidation that gets past vitamin E is supposed to be handled by glutathione. When vitamin E contacts an oxidant, such as hydrogen peroxide, it neutralizes it, but breaks into two parts in the process. That's the end of its antioxidant capacity, and a new molecule of vitamin E is needed to neutralize the next oxidant molecule that comes along. The vitamin E-oxidation product is detoxified by combination with glucuronic acid and excreted via bile. That's why our bodies need a good tocopherol supply when there is oxidant stress.

Antioxidant team members specialize to a great extent, and we need all of them to get the job done right.

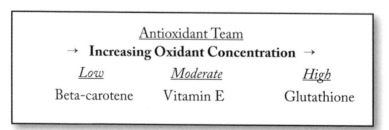

Selenium, at nutritional levels, is considered to be a sparing nutrient for vitamin E. That's because selenium (Se) is part of the glutathione peroxidase enzyme that facilitates glutathione's antioxidant activity.

$$2\ GSH + active\ oxidant \xrightarrow{\text{Se enzyme}} GSSG + neutralized\ oxidant$$

The more oxidants that GSH can handle, the less destruction there is of vitamin E. But in many with ASD, there's too little GSH and too much GSSG (oxidized glutathione).

NADPH is what gets GSH back from GSSG. Vitamin D helps NADPH formation; thiamine is required for it.

Antioxidant nutrients work as a team. Some years ago, the anti-vitamin cadre endeavored to prove that vitamin E supplementation alone is not beneficial. They did so. But as you know, a football player cannot score against an opposing team when there's not a team on his side to assist him. Cars don't move well with only one wheel, either, and a ladder with only one rung doesn't let you climb very far. Successful nutritional intervention requires teamwork, not a prima donna supplement. Please remember that when you visit the Internet or nutritional product vendors at meetings or conferences and when you visit health food stores.

Literature – Vitamins

National Research Council, Recommended Dietary Allowances, 10th Ed, Nat. Acad Press, Wash DC 1989

Shils, Olsen and Shike Modern Nutrition in Health and Disease, Lea & Febiger, multiple editions, 1990s

Kutsky R Handbook of Vitamins, Mineals and Hormones Van Norstrand Reinhold (1981)

Ames BN et al. "High-dose vitamin therapy stimulates variant enzymes…" Am J Clin Nutr 75 (4) Apr 2002, 606-58

Calabrese EJ Nutrition and Environmental Health, Vol. 1 The Vitamins, John Wiley & Sons, Wiley-Interscience, 1980

Chung JW et al. "Vitamin D_3 upregulated protein 1 (VDuP1) is a regulator for redox signaling and stress-mediated diseases" J Dermatol 33 (2006) 662-69

PDR for Nutritional Supplements, Thomson PDR, 1st Ed

Drug Facts and Comparisons, Wolters Kluwer Health, St. Louis MO (your pharmacist probably has this)

Levine M "New concepts in the biology and biochemistry of ascorbic acid" New Eng J Med 324 no.14 (Apr 3, 1986) 892-902

Lewin S Vitamin C: Its Molecular Biology and Medical Potential, Academic Press (1976)

Jacob R "Vitamin C" Chapt. 27 in Shils, Olson and Shike, Eds, Modern Nutrition in Health and Disease 8th Ed. Lea & Febiger (1994)

Rimland B "Vitamin C in the prevention and treatment of autism", Autism Research Review International, vol. 12, no2 (1998), ARI, San Diego. (While I take issue with the megadose levels mentioned, this is an interesting article by Dr. Rimland).

Rebec G, Centors J et al. "Ascorbic acid and the behavioral response to haloperidol: implications for the action of antipsychotic drugs" Science 227 (25 Jan 1985) 438-40.

SUPPLEMENT PRODUCTS TO BE WARY OF

N-acetylcysteine (NAC)

This can be a wonderful starter for glutathione synthesis, as it provides the needed but limiting amino acid cysteine. NAC has two commonly encountered drawbacks. (1) Often the material as provided is oxidized to some extent, and oxidized NAC simply adds to the tissue oxidant load. A pharmacy certifying NAC quality is a preferred source. (2) Regardless of the state of oxidation, NAC is a culture material for (intestinal) yeast growth, especially candida. If you choose to try NAC, also use antiyeast/fungal supplements such as octocosanol, olive leaf extract, and maybe Saccharomyces boulardii if yeast growth is suspected or confirmed (by stool analysis or urine biomarkers).

S-Adenosylmethionine (SAM or SAMe)

This one has been tried by several hundred parents per reports to ARI. It causes problems in almost as many as it helps, and the help is less than one-in-four. Based on now-known biochemistry, we don't want to use it if adenosine is above normal levels or when methylation is impaired, and these are significant problems for many with ASD. Supplemented SAM just adds to the burden of material that gets trapped by poorly-functioning metabolism.

Alpha-Lipoic Acid

This is sometimes suggested as an aid for detoxication or for mitochondrial function; lipoate is part of the pyruvate dehydrogenase complex which prepares chemical fuel for the citric acid cycle. The same cautions as for NAC apply here – oxidized material is counterproductive and intestinal yeast overgrowth is a threat.

Cycloserine

This actually is a prescription drug that sounds like an amino acid supplement. It's sometimes used to treat tuberculosis, because it inhibits growth of the mycobacterium. Parents occasionally ask about it. I believe cycloserine was proposed for autism because it also interacts with a neuronal receptor (NMDA) and may help neuronal synchrony and learning. However, it has undesirable actions including increasing the need for vitamin

B_6 as P5P and slowing down an enzyme that balances levels of glycine and serine. When serine becomes glycine, methylene tetrahydrofolate is made, which may sound like a good idea, but often isn't. It can result in more trapped 5-methylTHF (see folic acid in Vitamin chapter). It can also lead to more glycine, glyoxalate and oxalate. In some cases, it decreases vitamin B_{12} activity. This one is a double-edged sword and I don't like those things in autism; they often cut the wrong way.

Cysteine

It's too reactive and is prime culture material for candida. Don't use it as a stand-alone supplement. (It doesn't smell or taste good either!)

Cystine

I also don't recommend use of this as a stand-alone supplement. Like cysteine, it's a yeast-grower and it's the oxidized form of cysteine.

5-Hydroxytryptophan (5HTP)

5-HTP became available some years ago when tryptophan was banned by the FDA. This compound is what tryptophan becomes before it is made into serotonin. In due course, serotonin becomes melatonin. Don't use 5HTP until after you've addressed dysbiotic gut flora (after Tier 2). 5HTP used before this can increase dysbiosis and toxicant generation in the gut. Based on parent responses to ARI, 5HTP helps 47%, hinders 11%, and has no discernible effect for 42% (n=644, 2009).

Methylsulfonylmethane (MSM)

Despite its name, it doesn't help SAM methylation. It has been used on animals (mostly horses) to reduce oxidant stress that occurs with physical exertion. However, a published 2006 study on two human children reported a suspicious brain-wave abnormality attributed to regular ingestion of MSM (Willemsen et al., *Neuropediatrics* 37, 2006, 312-14). Brien et al. reviewed MSM and said that more scientific studies are needed to decide about MSM's possible benefits. (Brien S et al., *Osteoarth Cartilage* 16 (2008) 1277-88.) My conclusion – don't use it.

GLOSSARY AND ADDITIONAL INFORMATION

Adenosine, AMP, ADP, ATP

Adenosine is a molecule assembled inside body cells from parts of amino acids (glycine, glutamine, aspartic acid), from sugar (phosphorylated ribose), and from one-carbon chemical parts donated by forms of folic acid. The fancy name in biochemistry for molecules like adenosine is "purine nucleoside". Adenosine becomes a chemical energy transfer agent when it is loaded with phosphate: AMP (monophosphate), ADP (diphosphate), ATP (triphosphate – the highest energy form). When phosphate departs, released energy may be used to push a chemical change that would not otherwise occur. Often, adenosine becomes a major participant in the chemistry. For example, when ATP contacts methionine (in the presence of an enzyme that facilitates adenosyl transfer), the result is formation of S-adenosylmethionine, SAM. S stands for sulfur, the atom in methionine to which adenosine is attached. Once activated with its attached adenosine, SAM can give away its methyl part, provided that there's another kind of enzyme available to assist (transmethylase enzyme). Also, adenosine functions as a subunit of ribonucleic acid (RNA), and without its sugar and phosphorus, we know it as adenine, one of the four bases of DNA.

Acting as a neurotransmitter under normal conditions, adenosine has a calming effect. When adenosine is elevated, one consequence is decreased methylation, possibly leading to loss of neuronal synchrony. When adenosine isn't efficiently converted into other purine nucleosides (such as inosine), immune dysregulation can result.

There are forms of autism that feature abnormal metabolism of adenosine. A rare genetic form results from dysfunction of the enzyme adenylosuccinate lyase. Adenosine deaminase is another important enzyme; it promotes removal of nitrogen (amine part) of adenosine to form inosine. We do not have evidence that adenosine deaminase is dysfunctional in autism, but we do have evidence that a supporting protein is a problem for some. That supporting protein is dipeptidylpeptidase IV (DPP4), which holds some adenosine deaminase in place at the cell membrane. In an entirely different place, the mucosa of the small intestine, DPP4 is supposed to digest certain peptides from casein (dairy) and gluten (cereal grains). Per clinical studies by Karl Reichelt and others, DPP4 isn't getting that job done for many with autism. Direct evidence of something being wrong with adenosine comes from S. Jill James and others who report that 20% of autistic children have elevated blood plasma levels

163

of adenosine. The first clinical evidence of abnormal adenosine metabolism in autism was characterized by Gene Stubbs, et al, *J. Am Acad Child Psych* 21 (1982) 71-74.

Bioavailable or Bioavailability

This is a qualitative term that refers to how easy or how hard it is for the gastrointestinal tract to absorb a nutrient, especially a nutritional supplement. Substances that are water-soluble usually are quite bioavailable; calcium citrate is an example. Substances that are acid soluble are less bioavailable; calcium carbonate is an example. Some substances are just bio-unavailable because they are difficult to dissolve to form ions that can pass through the mucosal tissue; silicon dioxide or silica is an example. Once formed in the intestines, calcium oxalate is virtually insoluble and not bioavailable. Dietary fats and oils become bioavailable when the lipase enzyme and biliary function are working. So, bioavailablity depends upon the chemistry of the nutrient and upon the digestive capabilities of the individual.

Biopterin

This molecule is assembled in our cells to be a hydrogen-transferring cofactor. In its fully activated (chemically reduced) form, it carries four hydrogen atoms and is called tetrahydrobiopterin. In chemical reactions in our metabolism, it gives away two hydrogens to become dihydrobiopterin; then it needs a fillup of two hydrogen atoms to become activated again. The fillup comes from the top-grade reducing agent (hydrogen carrier) NADPH. Tetrahydrobiopterin is the necessary, hydrogen-providing cofactor for tryptophan to become 5-HTP, which becomes serotonin. It also is needed for phenylalanine to become tyrosine. Tyrosine is used to make thyroid hormones, dopamine, and other neurotransmitter amines.

Biopterin deficiency has been proposed for some with autism, particularly those with phenylalanine, tyrosine and tryptophan metabolism disorders. Orally-given tetrahydrobiopterin and biopterin have been used experimentally, but are expensive and relatively large oral amounts are needed. Comparatively few individuals with ASD have been significantly helped per information that I've seen. Spinal administration of tetrahydrobiopterin has shown promise and is reported on by Danfors et al., *J Clin Pharmacol* 25 no5 (2005) 485-89.

Bromine, brominated

Bromine is an element with chemistry similar to that of chlorine; brominated simply means that a chemical substance has had bromine added to it in chemical combination. Brominated chemicals are present in some flame retardants, fumigant sprays and sanitizing products. Flame retardants are used in many textile products including bedding and children's nightclothes. Polybrominated biphenyls (PBBs) are something it is best to avoid. These are 'organobromines" and they are first cousins to organochlorines.

Casein, casomorphins

Casein is part of the protein fraction of milk; how big a part depends upon which specie of animal we're concerned with. Here in the US we're concerned with Holstein (Friesian in the UK) cow milk versus human milk. Cow milk is 3.5% protein by weight; human milk is 1.1% protein by weight. Cow milk protein is 85% casein, 15% lactalbumin; human milk protein is 40% casein, 60% lactalbumin. Do the math and you'll find that a human infant has to contend with almost 7x as much casein when he/she drinks cow's milk as opposed to Mom's product. Further, casein is not exactly the same in amino acid sequence as we go from one animal to another. I'm told by experts that we may have made a mistake when we (the US) based its milk supply on the big black-and-white Holsteins instead of the smaller Jerseys or Guernseys. Holsteins produce more milk, but it's harder to digest.

A part of cow's casein, beta-casein, contains a short sequence of amino acids, beta-caso-morphins, that require dipeptidylpeptidase IV (DPP4) for digestion. With good DPP4, we'd still be okay. But then comes mistake #2 – exposure to mercury or organophosphates. Both (and some other toxicants as well) can knock out DPP4. The result is uptake of caso-morphin peptides into the bloodstream. Karl Reichelt and others have published a number of clinical studies showing presence of these peptides in many children with autism. An in vitro study shows immune dysregulation and other resulting problems – Vojdani et al., *Int J Immunopath Pharmacol* 16 (2003) 189-99

Chlorine, chlorinated

Chlorine is an element that combines readily with many other elements and with many chemical substances. Sometimes this produces a more active chemical substance or a chlo-rinated chemical that can oxidize other substances. Chlorinated simply means that the substance has one or more atoms of chlorine in its chemical makeup. For environmental toxiciology and the study of ASD, a major concern is chlorinated organic chemicals that are present and that a pregnant woman, fetus, or infant/child might encounter. The pesticides DDT, Dicofol, and endosulfan are examples. Please refer to the Background chapter for more information. Also see the Appendix for other examples of organochlorine toxicants.

Citric acid cycle

This is a cyclic (constantly repeating) chemical process that occurs in protected cellular compartments called mitochondria. A principal constituent of the cyclic process is citric acid. The process uses chemical fuel that's made primarily from dietary fats and carbohy-drates. The fuel-making process is internal to mitochondria for fats. This requires L-carni-tine and a process called "beta-oxidation", in which large fatty acid molecules are broken down into fuel-size pieces (a two-carbon chemical attached to coenzyme A called acetyl coenzyme A). For carbohydrates, most of the fuel-making occurs outside mitochondria and consists of breaking sugars down to the three-carbon acid called pyruvic acid or "pyruvate". Pyruvate is allowed into mitochondria where an enzyme system (pyruvate dehydrogenase) makes acetylCoA from it. The pyruvate-to-acetylCoA enzyme process requires coenzyme forms of vitamins B_1, B_2 and B_3 plus lipoic acid, and it can be impaired by some elemental toxicants (arsenic, mercury) and by various toxicant chemicals. Elevated blood pyruvate, indicating some hangup in pyruvate processing, has been reported for some with autism/ASD.

Amino acids also can be used to make pyruvate. When this happens, the cells have to be able to safely dispose of nitrogen. If they can't, ammonia excess will result – as it may for a marathon runner whose fat and carbohydrate reserves have been exhausted. Excess ammonia in cells and tissues can be toxic and life-threatening in extreme cases. Mildly elevated ammonia is sometimes identified in those with autism. When there is no evidence of infection, dysbiosis, or urea-cycle problems, elevated ammonia is suggestive of mito-chondrial dysfunction.

The citric acid cycle itself produces bicarbonate for acid-base balancing in body tissues and organs, and it generates hydrogen. The hydrogen participates in another chemical energy transfer process adjacent to the citric acid cycle, and that process enables the addition of phosphate to adenosine, eventually forming ATP. Those wishing to learn more about the citric acid cycle may do so by referring to any edition of Harper's Biochemistry, Lange Medical Publications. The citric acid cycle is also called the Krebs cycle in honor of the British scientist, H.A. Krebs, who postulated its chemistry in 1937 (he called it "citric acid cycle"). It's also called the tricarboxylic acid cycle.

Coenzyme

Some enzymes require a helper to promote chemical change. Many of these helpers are present in vitamin form in food, and they must be biochemically converted from vitamins to active coenzyme forms to be useful. Pyridoxine or vitamin B_6, for example, is transformed in cells to the coenzyme, pyridoxal 5-phosphate, "P5P". P5P gets attached to the enzyme-to-be, and once it's in place, the combination is ready to do its work. In the chemical process industry, enzymes would be called catalysts – they promote and/or accelerate otherwise non-occurring or slow chemical changes. Please refer to the first part of the Vitamin chapter for more information.

Cofactor

A cofactor is a substance that's needed, in addition to an enzyme, to make a chemical change or chemical reaction take place. A cofactor can be a coenzyme. It can also be something that provides a small but essential ingredient such as tetrahydrobiopterin providing hydrogen. Unlike an enzyme/coenzyme, which is left unchanged by the chemical reaction, some cofactors (e.g., biopterin) have to be regenerated before they can assist the next time. In this example, NADPH can also be considered a cofactor because it provides biopterin with replacement hydrogen.

Cytidine, CMP, CDP, CTP

Cytidine, like adenosine, has high-energy phosphate forms; it is a nucleoside composed of cytosine and ribose sugar. Cytidine is made differently, has a different chemical structure, and it gets its phosphates from ATP. CTP (or ATP) is needed to make coenzyme A from the vitamin pantothenic acid. CoA is required for numerous cell and tissue functions including mitochondrial energy processes. In DNA cytosine links with guanine. Cytosine is methylated or not to suppress or express genetic character. CTP, CDP and CMP are used to form phosphatidyl ethanolamine which, after methylation, becomes choline. Choline, in turn, forms betaine or TMG; TMG forms DMG – refer to the DMG/TMG chapters in this book for more information.

Cytosol, Cytosolic

This refers to the water-soluble part of a cell. It's the part that's partitioned off by fatty-acid membranes from the included compartments, such as the nucleus and mitochondria.

Activation of amino acids, fatty acid synthesis, and sugar chemistry (glycolysis, gluconeo-genesis) all take place in the cytosol. Also occurring in the cytosol is the methylTHF-cobalamin-homocysteine-to-methionine remethylation process.

Enzyme

An enzyme is a protein or protein complex that enables a chemical change in cells or in tissues (extracellular). For more information, please refer to the first part of the Vitamin chapter.

Fluoroquinolone

This refers to a class of substances that have antibiotic medication properties. They have similar chemical makeup – that being fluorine-containing organics that include a quinolone structure. Details of the chemistry are beyond the scope of this book but may be found online at PubChem using fluoroquinolones as a search term. A strain of the bacterium Clostridium difficile has developed resistance to fluoroquinolones, including ciprofloxacin, levofloxacin and others – Spigaglia et al. *J Med Microbiol* 57 (6) 2008 784-89. Other published research is confirming, see Saxton et al. *Antimicrob Agents Chemotherapy* 53 (2) 2009 412-20. This study suggests that fluoroquinolones actually encourage C. difficile infection.

FMN, FAD

These are abbreviations for two coenzyme (cofactor) forms of riboflavin, vitamin B_2. Please refer to the Vitamin chapter, riboflavin section, for further information.

Gluten

This is the general term for the large protein in wheat and other cereal grains that gives dough its resilient-elastic property. Part of gluten is gliadin, sometimes referred to as a protein, but more correctly it's a peptide piece of gluten. Included in gliadin is an amino acid sequence considered to be responsible for celiac disease. While wheat gluten/gliadin is the type often used to typify cereal grain protein, there are some differences in the amino acid sequences of gluten from wheat, rye, barley, oats, spelt, etc. Overall, these differences are minor. Like casein, incomplete digestion of all cereal grain glutens can lead to production of small peptides, which have opioid activities, inhibit enzymes (adenylate cyclase), and evoke immune responses in some individuals. Clinical studies by Reichelt and others have noted the presence of such peptides ("exorphins") in the urine of autistic children. Multiple, small-scale clinical studies have shown improvements for some with ASD in traits and behaviors, learning ability and decreased seizures after being on gluten- and casein-free diets for an extended period of time (months).

If you wish to pursue this, here are eight articles on the topic including a critical review from the Cochrane Database.

Reichelt, KL, Ekrem J et al. "Gluten, milk proteins and autism: dietary intervention effects on childhood autism" *J Appl Nutr* 1990, 42:1-22

Knivsberg A-M, Wilg K et al. "Dietary intervention in autistic syndromes" *Brain Dysfunction* 1990; 3: 315-27

Knivsberg A-M, Reichelt KL et al. "Autistic syndromes and diet: a follow-up study" *Scand J Educat Res* 1995; 39:223-36

Lucarelli S, Frediani T et al. "Food allergy and infantile autism" *Panminerva Med.* 1995; 37:137-41

Whitley P, Rodgers J et al. "A gluten-free diet as an intervention in autistic syndromes" *Autism* 1999:3:45-65

Knivsberg A-M, Reichelt KL et al. "A randomized controlled study of dietary intervention in autistic syndromes" *Nutr Neurosci.* 2002; 5:261-61

Millward C, Ferriter M et al. "Gluten and casein-free diets for autistic spectrum disorder " *Cochrane Database of Systematic Reviews* 2004, Issue 2, Art. No.: CD003498. DOI: 10.1002/14651858.pub2.

Whiteley P, Haracopos D et al. "The ScanBrit randomized, controlled, single-blind study of a gluten and casein-free dietary intervention for children with autism spectrum disorders' *Nutr. Neurosci.* 2010; 13:1-14

Guanosine, GMP, GDP, GTP

Guanosine is made by the same metabolic purine assembly line as adenosine. The only difference is the location of the nitrogen (amine) part on the molecule. The phosphates needed for GMP, GDP, GTP are supplied by ATP. Neuronal communication requires signal transfer, some of which involves the "G protein". When the G protein works, GTP goes to GDP (one phosphate is released) and the corresponding energy release is used to activate an enzyme or open a channel in a cell membrane to allow passage of ions (one step in signal transmission). Before it can work again, ATP has to replenish G's phosphate. After it does so, the resulting ADP needs its third phosphate back – phosphocreatine is hopefully close by and will provide it.

G-protein signal transmission is especially important for processing sensory inputs of vision (light), smell, and for alarm signals (epinephrine or adrenalin). GTP and G-protein involvement in autism is controversial. Some possibly pertinent issues include: (1) G protein function is disrupted by bacterial toxins; (2) synthesis of biopterin starts with GTP; (3) amounts of ATP are reduced in autistic brain (Minshew et al. Biol Pysch 33 (1993) 762-73), so GTP is likely to be limited as well. (4) Autistic traits and seizures may be present when creatine metabolism is disordered and neuronal phosphocreatine is deficient. One doctor who has investigated a possible autism link to G-protein function is Mary Megson, MD, *Med Hypotheses* 54 (6) 2000 979-83.

Hydroxylated

This means that a biochemical has been altered by addition of what chemists call a hydroxyl group, oxygen plus hydrogen, OH, and an electron. Adding OH with an electron can make a biochemical more stable, less reactive, and can be a step in detoxication. Benzene is very poisonous. Adding an OH makes it into phenol which isn't great but is a lot better than benzene. Phenylalanine, an essential amino acid, carries a benzene part. If it's not used for protein formation, one of the first things the body does with it is hydroxylate it. Phenylalanine with -OH on the benzene part is tyrosine and then it's ready to do something nice, like make thyroid hormones.

Methyl, methyl piece or group

The principal ingredient of natural gas is methane. Chemically, methane is a carbon atom with four attached hydrogen atoms. Methane is found throughout our solar system, throughout the universe as far as we know, and life here on earth evolved in the presence of it. So, it's not surprising that a whole lot of our biochemistry involves a chemically-active form of methane called a methyl group or simply "methyl". A carbon atom has four attachment points, something that's set by its outer shell of electrons. Methane uses all of them to hold four hydrogen atoms. When one hydrogen is removed from methane, the result is a methyl group with a vacant linkage point that can be used for attachment to something. A methyl is depicted as $-CH_3$. A carbon atom with an unused linkage can have a lot of companions instead a hydrogen atom, and a general name for this classification of chemical pieces is "one-carbon group" (see below). For many with autism, the exchange of methyls is disordered in their biochemistry.

Methylation, methylated

Our food provides methyls and our metabolism includes lots of methyl exchanges. Methionine and choline, both essential nutrients, and the nonessential amino acid glycine are all big nutrient sources of methyls. The process of adding methyl to a biochemical is "methylation", and enzymes that promote methyl exchanges among biochemicals are usually called methyl transferases. Methionine synthase is an exception; it promotes methyl exchange from methylated vitamin B_{12} to homocysteine to re-make some methionine. The B_{12} gets the methyl from tetrahydrofolate that might have gotten it from glycine.

When a biochemical is methylated, its personality and function typically are changed. Methylating the hormone serotonin makes something that acts differently – melatonin. Methylation of amino acids is a step in the assembly of creatine, L-carnitine, and internally-made choline. Methylation of fatty acids (or phospholipids) makes them more flexible, something that's essential for proper function of the cell membranes of neurons. Neurons with under-methylated membranes can't synchronize with each other, causing scrambled perception and response to sensory inputs. Methylation of cytosine in cytosine-guanosine (CG) pairs on DNA sets genetic expression and patterns of methylation are heritable – passed on from parents to offspring. Under-methylation corresponds to increased gene sensitivity/activity; and normal methylation maintains control of gene activity; overmethylation suppresses genetic expression.

Many individuals with autism feature impaired methylation; sometimes this is associated with increased adenosine. However, it isn't correct to say that the entire spectrum of methylation is subnormal in these individuals because there can be local areas of increased DNA methylation with gene suppression. Most of the methylation we're concerned with occurs via S-adenosylmethionine (SAM) giving away its methyl to form S-adenosylhomocysteine. A significant portion of the biochemical problems humans contend with is due to misadventures of S-adenosylhomocysteine metabolism caused by combinations of toxicants, infections and genetic imperfections.

Mitochondrion[s], Mitochondria[pl],

Most of the cells in our bodies (not red blood cells) contain protected compartments where sensitive biochemistry is carried out. A mitochondrial compartment or mitochondrion is double-walled by fatty-acid membranes and has monitored passageways in and out. Disassembly of fatty acids for cellular energy use, the citric acid cycle for hydrogen generation, and the respiratory chain that uses hydrogen and generates ATP all take place inside mitochondria. Some of the biochemical problems seen in autistic individuals, per laboratory analysis of blood and urine, are consistent with mitochondrial dysfunctions. These problems include: inadequate L-carnitine, pyruvate excess, and abnormalities among the chemical members of the citric acid cycle.

NAD, NADH, NADPH

These are coenzyme or cofactor forms of vitamin B_3, niacin. Please refer to the niacin section of the Vitamin chapter for more information.

One-carbon piece, one-carbon group

These are small chemical pieces, based on carbon, which get traded around by carrier molecules such as folate. When attached to the carrier molecule, they provide a distinct character to that molecule, allowing it to service a certain part of metabolism. Various one-carbon groups are shown in the Vitamin chapter, folic acid section. A methyl group (see above) is an example. Tetrahydrofolate carrying a formyl group can donate it to the purine assembly line. Without that, there's no formation of adenosine or guanosine. Tetrahydrofolate carrying methylene to the cytidine-uridine assembly line adjusts those quantities, and deficiency of methylene tetrahydrofolate is a possible reason for Fragile X syndrome. Unfortunately, if one-carbon transfers don't work right during fetal development, supplementing the missing substance after birth doesn't correct the condition.

Organic Acids

These are acid-acting chemicals based on carbon rather than fluorine, chlorine, bromine, iodine, sulfur, etc. The simplest one is formic acid, $HCOOH$; ants make it and you feel its sting when they bite. The $COOH$ part is the acid-acting part. CH_3COOH is the next biggest one; it's acetic acid and it's in vinegar. Acids donate a proton (a hydrogen ion) when they ionize – $CH_3COO^- + H^+$. Propionic acid (CH_3CH_2COOH) comes next in size and that's the one that produces autistic symptoms in rats per the studies of Dr. Derrick MacFabe et al. at the U of Western Ontario. It's also something that Clostridia make from amino acids; it's supposed to be cleared out of mitochondria by L-carnitine. If not, it becomes methylmalonic acid (MMA), and a B_{12}-dependent enzyme changes the MMA into the citric acid cycle chemical succinyl CoA. Please refer to the Vitamin B_{12} section of the Vitamin chapter for more information.

Oxalate

Internally, this is an end-stage substance from glycine metabolism. Externally it is a component of many foods (spinach, chard, rhubarb, chocolate, others). Internally, oxalate may be formed when the biochemistry of glycine is disordered. This can be a threat in autism if there is a one-carbon (methylene) transfer problem. Insufficient vitamin B_6 as P5P also is a risk factor for oxalate excess. Too much oxalate allows formation of insoluble calcium oxalate "stones" that may impair kidney function. Laboratory testing of blood/urine oxalate levels is offered by many clinical laboratories. Specimens should be tested promptly for accurate results; follow the lab's instructions precisely.

Dietary oxalate can be a problem when intestinal fat levels are high, as may occur with taurine, bile, or lipase enzyme insufficiencies. Fat in the intestines ties up calcium, allowing oxalic acid to be available for transport into the bloodstream. Adequate free calcium in the intestines combines with oxalic acid, making it insoluble and unabsorbable as calcium oxalate, and that oxalate is removed with fecal matter.

P5P

This is the coenzyme form of vitamin B_6, pyridoxine. Please refer to that section of the vitamin chapter for more information.

Purine

The purine assembly line is the biochemical sequence that makes adenosine and guanosine. Faults in this sequence have been proposed for autism, but confirmed cases of autism with disordered purine synthesis are unusual-to-rare. Contrary to this, problems with already-made adenosine seem to be common and could be present in 20 to 25% of autistic children. Those with adenosine problems and those with uric acid problems were once grouped as having "purine" autism. Uric acid is the final waste product of purine (adenosine, guanosine) metabolism.

Sulfate, sulfation

Fully oxidized sulfur is sulfate, and it can be attached to atoms (calcium sulfate), inorganic chemicals (ammonium sulfate), and to organic chemicals such as phenols and steroidal hormones with phenolic parts (estrone and bile salts are examples). Sulfation can make a biochemical more water-soluble and easier to excrete. In autism, the phenolsulfotransferase process (putting sulfate on phenols) may be impaired per the studies of Rosemary Waring (*Dev Brain Dysfunct* 10 (1997) 40-43). Possibly contributing to this are hang-ups in the metabolism sequence leading from methionine and homocysteine via cysteine to sulfate.

TACA

The abbreviation for the organization: Talk about Curing Autism. Lots of useful information is available. www.tacanow.org, Lisa Ackerman, POB 12409 Newport Beach CA 92658-2409.

APPENDIX

Circadian Rhythm and Nutrients

Our bodies operate with a 24-hour rhythm that's naturally set by environmental factors, nutritional input, and genetics. This rhythm requires food (fuel), daily activity (mental and physical), rest, repair and trash collection (detoxication). Some of this can be quite disturbed in those with ASD. Perhaps the most obvious disturbance is sleep during which much of rest, repair, and detoxication is supposed to take place. I consider immune defense to be mostly akin to these nighttime functions. You can help to normalize the circadian rhythm by matching some activities and supplements to the daily clock.

6:00-8:00 AM: Melatonin formation/secretion ceases, alertness increases, blood pressure increases, cells await new fuel supplies, amino acid stores need replenishment, digestion is ready to go. Breakfast happens – ideally, including high-quality protein. This is a good time for vitamin and amino acid supplements.

8:00-10:00 AM: Nutrients/fuel arrive in cells, where they're converted to energy for mental/physical functions. Tyrosine from protein and phenylalanine becomes dopamine (neuronal attention-getter) and is used to make thyroid hormones. Arginine and glycine get together to make the energy-delivery truck, creatine.

10:00AM-12:00 noon: A time of high mental alertness; it's good for relational therapy and special education. Cells are using up available fuel. Digestive needs are anticipated as noon approaches.

12:00 noon-2:00PM. Lunch happens. Feed with protein, carbs and fats. Cells get a fillup, but some temporary decrease in alertness is typical. A short rest period after lunch may be advisable. Supplements with lunch are fine; few restrictions apply at this time.

2:00-4:00PM. Cells are in peak performance mode. Mental reactions are fastest, hand-eye coordination is best. Another good time for interactive therapies.

4:00-6:00PM. Muscle strength peaks, then declines. Coordination and reaction time decrease. A meal with smaller protein and fat content is advisable as digestive capacities for these decreases. Cells are getting tired and are working less efficiently. Blood pressure rises. Antioxidant supplements such as vitamins C and E and some taurine go well at this time. Calcium and magnesium can also be supplemented with supper; also vitamin D.

6:00-7:00 PM. This is typically the time of highest body temperature and highest blood pressure. Cell energy conversion efficiency is down – they're tired. Zinc and calming nutrients go well at this time, including melatonin for young children who should go to sleep early. This can also be story time, but don't push questions or interactions now – you want sleep, not mental challenges.

7:00-10:00 PM. Tryptophan crosses blood-brain barrier, makes serotonin, serotonin makes melatonin and secretion of melatonin starts with decreased light exposure. Melatonin signals for cell regeneration materials including P5P from vitamin B_6, and melatonin acts to reduce inflammatory messengers (cytokines). Alertness declines and sleep begins. Cells assemble materials for cleaning and repair.

10:00PM-2:00AM. Sleep deepens and usually is deepest around 2:00 AM. Cell repair is underway. Melatonin secretion continues unless shut down by visual exposure to light.

2:00-5:00 AM. Body temperature reaches its lowest point, blood pressure is down and cells are either resting or finishing their rejuvenation activities. Wastes have been collected and put in urine or fecal matter. The first AM urination will contain a lot of evidence about cell function and metabolism.

5:00-6:00 AM. Melatonin secretion decreases, even before first light. Cells begin switching to receiving mode for outside news and eventual refueling (breakfast). Alertness begins.

6:00-8:00AM. The circadian cycle repeats.

Cooking with essential nutrients; nutrient stability

Because some children, especially young ones, can't or won't swallow capsules, one alternative strategy is to cook the contents into food. This poses a problem of destruction or partial destruction for some of the vitamins and a few other relatively fragile or easily-oxidized nutrients. Mixing the contents of supplement capsules with already-cooked food is far safer in terms of nutrient survival and for getting them into the intestinal tract. Nevertheless, for as many years as I can remember, moms have asked me about cooking with nutrients.

Minerals are mostly immune to cooking. They are elements and elements are chemical constants, at least for cooking activities. Calcium, zinc, magnesium, etc. stay as calcium, zinc and magnesium. And most of their supplemental forms – calcium as citrate or carbonate, zinc as citrate or complexed to amino acids, and magnesium as glycinate or citrate, survive as such at least up to 375°F. One that doesn't survive the oven very well is seleno-L-methionine; let's not cook with that one. Some mineral forms are quite refractory and you can't hurt them even with oven-cleaning temperatures (500°F): calcium carbonate, zinc oxide, magnesium oxide, also manganese and molybdenum oxides. The problem is, these forms aren't very bioavailable either – they're just very stable.

Chromium is a special case, and I advise not cooking with it at all. The biologically beneficial form, in trace amounts, is chromium with an oxidation state of +3 (CrIII). The bad chromium is oxidation state +6 (CrVI). Of course, all forms of chromium can be toxic at excessive levels. Baking CrIII can change it to toxic CrVI, so leave all chromium supplements out of cooking recipes.

Iodine is volatile and won't stay put during cooking, but the usual and safe supplement form is sodium or potassium iodide. These iodides are stable to way above kitchen oven temperatures.

Microwaving won't change an element either. But microwaving may change the element's attached organic molecules in undesirable ways. Microwave cooking differs from the thermal cooking that occurs in standard electric or gas-fired ovens. There, heat is transferred by convection and by radiation that extends into the infrared spectrum. Microwaves are a "higher" form of energy, i.e. electromagnetic energy with a frequency spectrum extending into the far infrared (300,000 to 300,000,000 Hertz). Microwaves dissipate the vast majority of their radiant energy as heat – but not necessarily all of it. Some microwave energy may be used to alter the chemical bonds (connections) between elements or parts of molecules in the food, resulting in chemical changes that may not be healthy –changing cis-to-trans configured oils/fats comes to mind. Microwaving definitely destroys vitamin B_{12} (Wantanabe, *J Agric Food Chem* __46__ (1) (1998) 206-10).

So microwave cooking is kind of an unknown, and I don't know if amino acid-chelated mineral supplements stay properly chelated when microwaved. Behavior of glutathione, L-carnitine, melatonin and other reactive or sensitive nutrients is likewise unknown in a microwave environment. My advice is to avoid microwaving foods that you've added any supplemental nutrients to.

Never cook digestive enzymes or probiotics. Digestive enzymes are mostly destroyed by cooking and little if any digestive function will survive. Microorganisms, including those in probiotics, whether dormant or not, will be killed quickly by microwaves. A capsule containing a billion colony forming units goes to less than measurable CFU in about 30 seconds.

Essential fatty acids are long-chain carbon molecules, and the carbon atoms within are naturally attached to each other in one of two ways, "cis" and "trans". In our bodies, metabolism works primarily with cis-configured fatty acids; trans fatty acids tend to clog up the works. That's why you see "no trans fatty acids" on some food labels today. Well, cooking cis-fatty acids for too long a time or especially at too high a temperature can change some of these to the trans configuration. So, don't include the fish oils and other cis-configured essential fatty acids in baking or cooking projects. And when you bake fish, baking for a long time at a low temperature is better than a shorter time at a high temperature.

Now, how about cooking vitamins? That has been the most-asked-about nutrient category, at least for me. The vitamins are all different; some are resistant and tough to harm by cooking or baking while others are fragile and easily destroyed. While we're on the topic, let's talk about exposure to air and light, particularly sunlight. Ultraviolet exposure is a killer for most vitamins. That's why they're packaged in opaque plastic [or glass] bottles.

Vitamin A – susceptible to oxidation in air, and is destroyed rapidly (hours) by exposure to sunlight. It begins to degrade at temperatures above 150°F, so you can't cook with vitamin A. Beta carotene is more stable, and baking or boiling yellow/orange vegetables like squash or carrots degrades only a small portion of it.

Vitamin B_1 (thiamine) is relatively stable in air but is destroyed by decomposition (breaks into chemical pieces) with ultraviolet (sunlight) exposure. Okay for cooking up to 400°F.

Vitamin B_2 (riboflavin) is susceptible to oxidation in air, and is rather quickly decomposed by ultraviolet exposure. It's okay for baking in food up to 350°F.

Vitamin B_3 is relatively air and light stable as niacin, and can be heated to 420°F. However, the niacinamide form should not be baked above 325°F.

Vitamin B_6 is more stable as pyridoxine.HCl, which oxidizes slowly in air and is okay up to 300°F. Pyridoxine and pyridoxal forms, including pyridoxal 5-phosphate, are less stable, are destroyed by ultraviolet exposure, and are less likely to survive cooking or baking.

Vitamin B_{12} is susceptible to oxidation in air and degradation by ultraviolet light. B_{12} can be heated or baked in food to about 360°F without destruction, provided the baking time at that temperature doesn't exceed one or two hours. This holds for cyanocobalamin supplements. Methylcobalamin data is lacking but it's known to be a much more fragile form of B_{12}. I suggest not cooking methylcobalamin.

Folic acid is susceptible to oxidation in air and degradation by exposure to ultraviolet light. Baking in food up to 375°F is okay for 1-2 hours.

Pantothenic acid is relatively stable in supplement forms such as calcium pantothenate, and it can be baked to 375°F.

Vitamin C is very susceptible to oxidation in air, and it is destroyed by ultraviolet light. Auto-oxidation (without oxygen) occurs with molecular changes catabolized by trace copper or iron (cooking utensil surfaces) at temperatures above 200°F. There is rapid degradation with oven baking above 200°F. Mostly, this one just doesn't survive cooking.

Vitamin D is susceptible to oxidation in air and is destroyed by ultraviolet exposure. It degrades at temperatures above 180°F, so this one's not for cooking either.

Vitamin E is very susceptible to oxidation in air and is destroyed by ultraviolet exposure. It degrades at temperatures above 275°F. Also, vitamin E doesn't do well in acidic foods, so don't expect it to survive blending or cooking with tomato/pasta sauce, citrus, pickles and vinegar-added foods, or kraut and "sour" foods. Vitamin C and E are antioxidants; that means they get oxidized while something more important doesn't. So, cooking these vitamins amounts to purposeful oxidation and is counterproductive.

Twenty Pesticides, Herbicides, Fungicides To Especially Avoid

Chemical/Example Common Names	Possible Effects[1]	Typical Exposure Sites
2,4-D (herbicide) "Barrage", "Bush Killer", "Campaign"; an organochlorine	neurotoxic, hepato-toxic, reproductive toxicant	farms, pastures, range-lands, forests, lawn & garden sprays
Alachlor (pre-emergence herbicide), "Lariat", "Lasso", an organo-chlorine	mutagenic	farms, field crops incl. corn, peanuts & soybeans
Bifenthrin (acaricide, insecticide), "Brigade", "Capture","Talstar",, organochlorine-fluorine	reproductive toxicant, neurotoxin	general agricultural use, lawn & garden, food crop residues
Captan (fungicide), many brand names, thiophthalimide organochlorine	mutagenic, fetal damage reported	general crop use; cancelled 1989, still used for apples, almonds, strawberries; might be on wallpaper, in paints, shipping crates
Chlorpyrifos (insecticide) "Dursban", "Lorsban", "Pilot", organochlorine phosphate	neurotoxic	general use, agriculture, commercial, residential, food crop residue
Diazinon (pesticide) Wide US use prior to 2001; general foreign Use persists organo-, phosphate	neurotoxic	restricted to agricultural uses, veterinary, licensed professionals, food crop residues
Dicofol (miticide & insecticide), "Difol", "Kelthane", organochlorine	neurotoxic; use correlated with autism incidence[2]	agricultural use, food crop residues, cotton, plant nur-series, ornamental plants
Diuron (herbicide) "Di-On", "Diumate", urea-organochlorine that inhibits photosynthesis	irritant, carcinogenic? fetal damage reported	General use for weeds, rangelands, food crop residues cotton, sugar cane
Endosulfan (insecticide, acaricide) "Endoside", Many brand names, cyclodiene-type organo chlorine	neurotoxic, use correlated with autism incidence[2]	agricultural use, food crop residues, now in process of being banned internationally

Twenty Pesticides, Herbicides, Fungicides To Especially Avoid

Chemical/Example Common Names	Possible Effects[1]	Typical Exposure Sites
Fenitrothion (acaricide, insecticide), "Cytel", "Fenitox", "Metathion" "MED", organophosphate	neurotoxic	general use pesticide, mosquitos, flies, flour/grain beetles, locusts, rice, orchard fruits, cereals
Glyphosate (herbicide) "Roundup", "Campaign" "FieldMaster", organophosphate	recent studies show embryonic cell damage due to adjuvants and metabolites from commercial products[3]	farms, rangelands, lawn and garden, forests, parks, food crop residues
Hexachlorophene (fungicide) "Hexafen", "G-Eleven", organochlorine – chlorinated phenol type	neurotoxic, birth defects reported	agricultural use, citrus & some vegetables, in soaps, shampoos, deodorants
Malathion (insecticide) Many brand names incl. "All Purpose Garden insecticide"; organophosphate	neurotoxic, reproductive toxicant, personality changes reported	general use, agricultural, commercial and residential, food crop residues
MCPA (herbicide) "Agritox", "Borden-Master, "Cheyenne", organochlorine, chlorophenoxy type	reproductive toxicant, mutagenic?	farms, ranches, grasslands, food crop residues
Methoxychlor (insecticide) chemical relative of DDT w/over 800 brand names active + cancelled since 1945; organochlorine	reproductive toxicant, neurotoxic	registered use for >80 crops, food crop residues, drinking water contaminant
Phosmet (insecticide, acaricide) "Fireban", "Del-Phos", "APPA" organophosphate	highly toxic neurotoxin	fire ant control, pet collars, livestock areas, some food crop residues
Temephos (larvicide, insecticide) "Abate", "Abathion", organophosphate	neurotoxic	ponds, wetlands, for mosquito control

Twenty Pesticides, Herbicides, Fungicides To Especially Avoid

Chemical/Example Common Names	Possible Effects[1]	Typical Exposure Sites
Tetrachlorvinphos (insecticide) "Clean Crop", "Fly Patrol" organophosphate	neurotoxic	farms, ranches, feedlots poultry houses – applied dermally, pet collars, over 80 EPA-registered products
Thiophanate-methyl (fungicide, antihelmintic) "Cercobin", "Domain" "Fungitox", "Funga", benzimidazole type carbamate	male and female reproductive toxin, neurotoxic, hepato-toxic	greenhouses, plant nurseries fruit & vegetable crops, food crop residues
Trichlorfen (insecticide) Many product names organophosphate	neurotoxic, hepatoxic	pastures, lawns, golf courses, ornamental plants, plant nurseries. All food crop use cancelled in US, 1995

---

1. Possible effects of these chemicals include those of animal studies, because it is ethically impossible to test with human subjects. Many of these effects, however, are for humans with occupational or unintended exposures.
2. See Roberts EM et al, "Maternal residence near agricultural pesticide applications and autism spectrum disorders among children in the california central valley" *Environ Health Perspect* 115 (10) Oct 2007, 1482-89.
3. Benachour N and Seralini GE "Glyphosate formulations induce apoptosis and necrosis in human umbilical, embryonic and placental cells" *Chem Res Toxicol* 22 (1) Jan 2009, 97-105.

PARENT RATINGS OF BEHAVIORAL EFFECTS OF BIOMEDICAL INTERVENTIONS
Autism Research Institute • 4182 Adams Avenue • San Diego, CA 92116

The parents of autistic children represent a vast and important reservoir of information on the benefits—and adverse effects—of the large variety of drugs and other interventions that have been tried with their children. Since 1967 the Autism Research Institute has been collecting parent ratings of the usefulness of the many interventions tried on their autistic children.

The following data have been collected from the more than 27,000 parents who have completed our questionnaires designed to collect such information. For the purposes of the present table, the parents responses on a six-point scale have been combined into three categories: "made worse" (ratings 1 and 2), "no effect" (ratings 3 and 4), and "made better" (ratings 5 and 6). The "Better:Worse" column gives the number of children who "Got Better" for each one who "Got Worse."

DRUGS	Got Worse[A]	No Effect	Got Better	Better: Worse	No. of Cases[B]
Actos	19%	60%	21%	1.1:1	140
Aderall	43%	26%	31%	0.7:1	894
Amphetamine	47%	28%	25%	0.5:1	1355
Anafranil	32%	39%	29%	1.1:1	440
Antibiotics	33%	50%	18%	0.5:1	2507
Antifungals[C]					
Diflucan	5%	34%	62%	13:1	1214
Nystatin	5%	43%	52%	11:1	1969
Atarax	26%	53%	21%	0.8:1	543
Benadryl	24%	50%	26%	1.1:1	3230
Beta Blocker	18%	51%	31%	1.7:1	306
Buspar	29%	42%	28%	1.0:1	431
Chloral Hydrate	42%	39%	19%	0.5:1	498
Clonidine	22%	32%	46%	2.1:1	1658
Clozapine	38%	43%	19%	0.5:1	170
Cogentin	20%	53%	27%	1.4:1	198
Cylert	45%	35%	19%	0.4:1	634
Depakene[D]					
Behavior	25%	44%	31%	1.2:1	1146
Seizures	12%	33%	55%	4.6:1	761
Desipramine	34%	35%	32%	0.9:1	95

DRUGS	Got Worse[A]	No Effect	Got Better	Better: Worse	No. of Cases[B]
Dilantin[D]					
Behavior	28%	49%	23%	0.8:1	1127
Seizures	16%	37%	47%	3.0:1	454
Fenfluramine	21%	52%	27%	1.3:1	483
Haldol	38%	28%	34%	0.9:1	1222
IVIG	7%	39%	54%	7.6:1	142
Klonapin[D]					
Behavior	31%	40%	29%	0.9:1	270
Seizures	29%	55%	16%	0.6:1	86
Lithium	22%	48%	31%	1.4:1	515
Luvox	31%	37%	32%	1.0:1	251
Mellaril	29%	38%	33%	1.2:1	2108
Mysoline[D]					
Behavior	41%	46%	13%	0.3:1	156
Seizures	21%	55%	24%	1.1:1	85
Naltrexone	18%	49%	33%	1.8:1	350
Low Dose Naltrexone	11%	52%	38%	4.0:1	190
Paxil	34%	32%	35%	1.0:1	471
Phenobarb.[D]					
Behavior	48%	37%	16%	0.3:1	1125
Seizures	18%	44%	38%	2.2:1	543

DRUGS	Got Worse[A]	No Effect	Got Better	Better: Worse	No. of Cases[B]
Prolixin	30%	41%	28%	0.9:1	109
Prozac	33%	32%	35%	1.1:1	1391
Risperidal	21%	26%	54%	2.6:1	1216
Ritalin	45%	26%	29%	0.6:1	4256
Secretin					
Intravenous	7%	50%	43%	6.4:1	597
Transderm.	9%	56%	35%	3.9:1	257
Stelazine	29%	45%	26%	0.9:1	437
Steroids	34%	30%	36%	1.1:1	204
Tegretol[D]					
Behavior	25%	45%	30%	1.2:1	1556
Seizures	14%	33%	53%	3.8:1	872
Thorazine	36%	40%	24%	0.7:1	945
Tofranil	30%	38%	32%	1.1:1	785
Valium	35%	42%	24%	0.7:1	895
Valtrex	8%	42%	50%	6.7:1	238
Zarontin[D]					
Behavior	34%	48%	18%	0.5:1	164
Seizures	20%	55%	25%	1.2:1	125
Zoloft	35%	33%	31%	0.9:1	579

BIOMEDICAL/ NON-DRUG/ SUPPLEMENTS	Got Worse[A]	No Effect	Got Better	Better: Worse	No. of Cases[B]
Calcium[E]	3%	60%	36%	11:1	2832
Cod Liver Oil	4%	41%	55%	14:1	2550
Cod Liver Oil with Bethanecol	11%	53%	36%	3.4:1	203
Colostrum	6%	56%	38%	6.8:1	851
Detox. (Chelation)[C]	3%	23%	74%	24:1	1382
Digestive Enzymes	3%	35%	62%	19:1	2350
DMG	8%	50%	42%	5.3:1	6363
Fatty Acids	2%	39%	59%	31:1	1680
5 HTP	11%	42%	47%	4.2:1	644
Folic Acid	5%	50%	45%	10:1	2505
Food Allergy Trtmnt	2%	31%	67%	27:1	1294
Hyperbaric Oxygen Therapy	5%	30%	65%	12:1	219
Magnesium	6%	65%	29%	4.6:1	301
Melatonin	8%	26%	66%	8.3:1	1687
Methyl B12 (nasal)	10%	45%	44%	4.2:1	240
Methyl B12 (subcut.)	6%	22%	72%	12:1	899
MT Promoter	8%	47%	44%	5.5:1	99
P5P (Vit. B6)	11%	40%	48%	4.3:1	920
Pepcid	11%	57%	32%	2.9:1	220
SAMe	16%	62%	23%	1.4:1	244
St. Johns Wort	19%	64%	18%	0.9:1	217
TMG	16%	43%	41%	2.6:1	1132

BIOMEDICAL/ NON-DRUG/ SUPPLEMENTS	Got Worse[A]	No Effect	Got Better	Better: Worse	No. of Cases[B]
Transfer Factor	8%	47%	45%	5.9:1	274
Vitamin A	3%	54%	44%	16:1	1535
Vitamin B3	4%	51%	45%	10:1	1192
Vit. B6/Mag.	4%	46%	49%	11:1	7256
Vitamin C	2%	52%	46%	20:1	3077
Zinc	2%	44%	54%	24:1	2738

SPECIAL DIETS

	Got Worse[A]	No Effect	Got Better	Better: Worse	No. of Cases[B]
Candida Diet	3%	39%	58%	21:1	1141
Feingold Diet	2%	40%	58%	26:1	1041
Gluten- /Casein- Free Diet	3%	28%	69%	24:1	3593
Low Oxalate Diet	7%	43%	50%	6.8:1	164
Removed Chocolate	2%	46%	52%	28:1	2264
Removed Eggs	2%	53%	45%	20:1	1658
Removed Milk Products/Dairy	2%	44%	55%	32:1	6950
Removed Sugar	2%	46%	52%	27:1	4589
Removed Wheat	2%	43%	55%	30:1	4340
Rotation Diet	2%	43%	55%	23:1	1097
Specific Carbo- hydrate Diet	7%	22%	71%	10:1	537

A. "Worse" refers only to worse behavior. Drugs, but not nutrients, typically also cause physical problems if used long-term.
B. No. of cases is cumulative over several decades, so does not reflect current usage levels (e.g., Haldol is now seldom used).
C. Antifungal drugs and chelation are used selectively, where evidence indicates they are needed.
D. Seizure drugs: top line behavior effects, bottom line effects on seizures
E. Calcium effects are not due to dairy-free diet; statistics are similar for milk drinkers and non-milk drinkers.

INDEX

185